CW00434161

Blood Labs 3

A guide to interpreting blood test results for cardiovascular disease

This book is dedicated to:

Gillian Cohen and her purple hair bobble f*ckery which inadvertently helped me to start writing this book.

Debbie Grayson, whose support and mentoring is beyond compare.

And of course, to all my Bleeks, James, family, and friends – all of whom supported me with excuses to procrastinate just enough to keep me sane, but not enough to delay the book being written.

CONTENTS

FOREWORD

We all have internal bias. We are only human!

Weight bias is ingrained in our society. It is heavily influenced by both overt and covert messaging from the medical professions, the media, the fashion industry and the diet industry.

We receive so many messages about weight that we have to be exceptionally careful to check our bias regularly. We are less likely to make health judgements of a client who is underweight or 'normal' weight but excess weight can conjur up concepts of diet and lifestyle that may be inaccurate.

It is fundamental to being able to offer personalised and non-judgemental healthcare, that we understand that cholesterol dysregulation is not sizeist and can affect underweight, 'normal' weight, or overweight individuals. The same can and should be said about any dysregulation within the body.

Nicky Gregory
www.thefatnutritionaltherapist.com

MEDICAL DISCLAIMER

This book is not going to tell you whether you should take the statins you or your client have been prescribed.

This book is for nutritional therapists supporting their client's wellbeing and using blood tests to monitor their nutritional interventions.

This book is not aimed at the general public. That's not to say that you can't read this book if you're not a nutritional therapist, but you should do so at your own risk.

1. Credit
   a. This document was created using a template from Docular (https://docular.net).
2. No advice
   a. This book contains general medical information.
   b. The medical information is not advice and should not be treated as such.
3. No warranties
   a. The medical information in this book is provided without any representations or warranties, express or implied.
   b. Without limiting the scope of Section 3a, we do not warrant or represent that the medical information in this book:
      i. will be constantly available, or available at all; or
      ii. is true, accurate, complete, current, or non-misleading.
4. Medical assistance
   a. You must not rely on the information in this book as an alternative to medical advice from your doctor or other professional healthcare provider.
   b. If you have any specific questions about any medical matter, you should consult your doctor or other professional healthcare provider.
   c. If you think you may be suffering from any medical condition, you should seek immediate medical attention.
   d. You should never delay seeking medical advice, disregard medical advice or discontinue medical treatment because of information in this book.
5. Limits upon exclusions of liability
   a. Nothing in this disclaimer will:
      i. limit or exclude any liability for death or personal injury resulting from negligence;
      ii. limit or exclude any liability for fraud or fraudulent misrepresentation;
      iii. limit any liabilities in any way that is not permitted under applicable law; or
      iv. exclude any liabilities that may not be excluded under applicable law.

INTRODUCTION

"High cholesterol is the problem"

This is something I remember hearing when I was younger – my dad was diagnosed with high cholesterol and still, to this day, has regular blood tests to monitor his cholesterol levels.

I grew up nervous about even the word cholesterol and, despite never having been told I had a cholesterol issue, I would actively seek out the processed low-fat foods in shops to avoid developing high cholesterol myself.

When I became a nutritional therapist, I wasn't 100% sure how to advise my clients on their cholesterol levels and would quietly panic inside when asked for advice. Client's doctors were prescribing various statins, and I knew that it was outside my remit to advise against this. Supplement companies seemed to advertise a plethora of alternative solutions though – red yeast rice, plant sterols and plant stanols, probiotics – all seemingly aimed at lowering cholesterol.

But the nutritional therapist in me wasn't convinced that simply lowering cholesterol through supplements or medications, without addressing diet and lifestyle, was the complete solution. In fact, it sounded an awful lot like turning off the fire alarm but leaving the fire burning.

(You'll find that I have used a few analogies to explain complex ideas in this book – and I'm afraid you'll just have to get used to them!)

In college, I recalled that we were taught it was sugar, not fat, that raised cholesterol levels. Or perhaps inflammatory lifestyles. Or genetics. But all of this seemed to disagree with what I'd learnt growing up about cholesterol only being associated with saturated fat intake, and it left me feeling conflicted.

I'd read that the majority of cholesterol is produced in the liver rather than from dietary intake, which made me question my knowledge even further.

I'd heard of "happy" HDL and "lousy" LDL cholesterol, but not touched on triglycerides or ratios, or explored further into particle sizes. And I'd certainly not heard of apolipoproteins.

I first got my cholesterol tested as part of a "what's wrong with me?" MOT when I was aged 36 or so. At that point, I was 2 years into a low carbohydrate, unprocessed Paleo style diet, eating vegetables either steamed or cooked with coconut or extra virgin olive oil, served with meat or fish three times a day. My doctor was keen to test my cholesterol levels because of my family history and because of my diet, which she was adamant was akin to a death sentence for me. I was nervous because I loved the Paleo meals I was cooking and it had done wonders for my fatigue issues but, if I was honest, the old-school emphasis on saturated fat causing raised cholesterol was weighing heavy on my mind.

When the blood results came back my cholesterol results were a surprise to both of us. My total cholesterol was 3.5mmol/L and my LDL and HDL were both sitting at 1.7mmol/L each. I had a call with my doctor to discuss the overall results, and she refused to believe my diet could result in such low cholesterol levels.

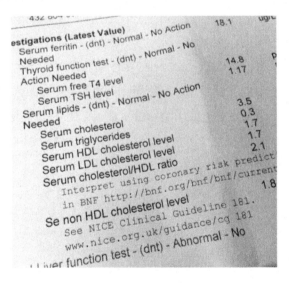

I was happy to see my results so low, and so was my doctor – in her opinion, we should always be aiming for total cholesterol and LDL cholesterol to be as low as possible. She made it sound like zero was the perfect number to aim for in terms of cholesterol.

Now though, having researched and written this book, I wonder if my cholesterol levels were maybe a little too low. If I saw a client with results like these now, I would question if they were eating enough, test their apolipoproteins and genetics in more detail, and explore whether the low production of cholesterol was impacting their cellular health, brain health, and production of other steroid hormones such as oestrogen and testosterone. Certainly, if there was any question over fertility, I would now look to increase their cholesterol level if it was below 4mmol/L.

Hopefully, reading this book will empower you with the skills and confidence to support your clients with nutritional interventions targeted at improving their cholesterol results when needed, and knowing how to seek reassurance regarding raised cholesterol levels. I know I'll be addressing my client's cholesterol reports differently going forwards!

Kate x

CHAPTER 1: CHOLESTEROL AND BUS NETWORKS

We may feel scared and panic a little when we hear of raised cholesterol because, for many years, there has been an association between raised cholesterol and clogged/furred arteries leading to health problems such as atherosclerotic cardiovascular disease – i.e. we've been told that excess cholesterol accumulates in arteries and causes blockages leading to heart attacks, strokes, and the need for a statin to be prescribed to improve those cholesterol levels. In essence, we've been told that raised cholesterol without a statin is a death sentence. Both the NHS and American Heart Association also list reducing fatty foods, exercising more, stopping smoking, and cutting down on alcohol as solutions for lowering cholesterol but (*in my best sarcastic voice*) who wants to do all of that when there's a magic pill that can do it for us?! I digress...

But the question that comes to my mind is: is raised cholesterol really the cause of atherosclerotic cardiovascular disease? Or is it the environment that the cholesterol is living in that leads to the atherosclerotic cardiovascular disease? Are the cholesterol levels a symptom, rather than a cause? Is cholesterol really the bad guy we've all been told?

Newer research is suggesting that the association between cholesterol levels and cardiovascular disease is not as simple as this, and that raised cholesterol isn't necessarily the death sentence that it has previously been seen as. Latest research is suggesting that there may be less association between cholesterol levels and atherosclerotic cardiovascular disease than previously thought and that lifestyle is as important as the cholesterol level itself.

Arteries carry the blood from the heart to the tissues and organs, while veins carry the blood back to the heart from the tissues, together with any waste products from the cells. This network of blood vessels is the body's vascular system. Nitric oxide is produced in the endothelial cells lining the vascular system and plays a strong role in the maintenance of vascular homeostasis – aka keeping the blood vessels healthy and maintaining adequate blood pressure. When certain lifestyle habits are adopted (e.g. smoking cigarettes, poor dietary choices, lack of exercise) or less nitric oxide is produced (often due to those same lifestyle habits, or from low vitamin D, or simply from ageing), these endothelial cells can become damaged, resulting in endothelial dysfunction.

Dr. Malcolm Kendrick, author of "The Clot Thickens" and "The Great Cholesterol Con" has researched endothelial dysfunction, cholesterol, and atherosclerotic cardiovascular disease extensively, and I highly recommend reading his books and/or reading his blogs on his website, as I could never consolidate all his research into one line, one page, or even one chapter, here.

Dyslipidaemia is recognised as the imbalance of lipoproteins because of dietary and lifestyle choices, or genetic predisposition, and may present as:

- Raised triglycerides
- Low HDL
- Normal or raised LDL

Now, let's go back to the basics to break this down and understand it better.

If you don't know your lipoproteins from your apolipoproteins, then this part of the chapter is for you.

In very simple terms, cholesterol is a waxy, fat-like substance. The majority of our cholesterol (70%) is endogenous or made in our livers. But cholesterol is also present in some foods that we eat – full fat dairy, coconut, shellfish, and red meat for example are sources of exogenous cholesterol, and exogenous cholesterol makes up approximately 30% of our cholesterol.

Cholesterol molecules form a key component of the phospholipid bilayer of cellular membranes, maintaining stability of the membrane itself and keeping the phospholipids together to allow selective passage of specific substances through the membrane. Without cholesterol, every cell would be floppy and leaky.

Cholesterol can be found in the nervous system, the brain, and the myelin sheath of nerves.

It is also a precursor to steroid and sex hormones – oestrogens, progestins, testosterone, cortisol, aldosterone, androgens; it forms an essential role in the hydroxylation of vitamin D3 from the skin or diet into calcidiol; and it is used in the synthesis of bile in the liver.

In short, we need cholesterol.

When we eat, any calories from the food consumed that are not required straight away will be broken down into their component fatty acids that are then grouped up into a chain of three fatty acids, with a molecule of glycerol holding them together. These are known as triglycerides.

Cholesterol and triglycerides are hydrophobic (insoluble) in the bloodstream, and therefore need to be transported through the bloodstream by something that is not hydrophobic.

Which leads us neatly on to the lipoproteins.

The lipoproteins have a hydrophilic membrane allowing them to travel through the bloodstream. They transport cholesterol and triglycerides which are safely tucked away in their hydrophobic cores. Lipoproteins are divided into seven classes based on their size, apolipoproteins (we'll come to those shortly), and lipid composition. The lipoproteins names are chylomicrons, chylomicron remnants, VLDL, IDL, LDL, HDL, and Lp(a).

Some of these lipoproteins are instantly recognisable as what we know as cholesterol markers in blood tests. Yes, this is confusing – LDL cholesterol and HDL cholesterol markers are lipoproteins but stick with me. If I can get my head around this, so can you.

All the lipoproteins have a similar structure, regardless of their size or lipid composition:

- Hydrophobic core containing cholesterol esters, triglycerides
- Hydrophilic phospholipid bilayer membrane featuring phospholipids, free cholesterol, apolipoproteins

Chylomicrons

These are formed in the intestines and carry dietary triglycerides and cholesterol to the peripheral tissues and the liver.

The size of chylomicrons will vary depending on the meal eaten – higher fat meals will result in an increase in the number of triglycerides produced, and subsequently larger sized chylomicrons to carry the triglycerides. When in a fasted state, chylomicrons are smaller due to lower levels of triglycerides.

Chylomicron Remnants

These are formed when triglycerides leave the chylomicron to enter peripheral tissues. Chylomicron remnants are therefore cholesterol-rich and triglyceride-poor.

Very Low-Density Lipoproteins VLDL

These are formed in the liver and their size varies depending on the quantity of triglycerides produced by the liver. An increase in production of triglycerides will result in an increased size of VLDL.

Intermediate Density Lipoproteins IDL

These are formed when triglycerides from VLDL enter muscle and adipose tissues, leaving IDL particles which are cholesterol rich.

Low-Density Lipoproteins LDL

These are derived from VLDL and IDL and carry the majority of the cholesterol in circulation. Their size varies from small and dense, to large and buoyant.

High-Density Lipoproteins HDL

These are formed in the liver and collect cholesterol from the peripheral tissues, transporting it back to the liver for recycling/elimination via bile. HDL is also anti-inflammatory and has antioxidant properties.

Lp(a)

These are made in the liver and carry triglycerides, similar to LDL.

This table neatly summarises the differences of the lipoproteins, in terms of size, density, lipids, and apolipoproteins:

Lipoprotein	Density (g/ml)	Size (nm)	Major Lipids	Major Apolipoproteins
Chylomicrons	<0.930	75-1200	Triglycerides	Apo B-48, Apo C, Apo E, Apo A-I, A-II, A-IV
Chylomicron Remnants	0.930- 1.006	30-80	Triglycerides & Cholesterol	Apo B-48, Apo E
VLDL	0.930- 1.006	30-80	Triglycerides	Apo B-100, Apo E, Apo C
IDL	1.006- 1.019	25-35	Triglycerides & Cholesterol	Apo B-100, Apo E, Apo C
LDL	1.019- 1.063	18- 25	Cholesterol	Apo B-100
HDL	1.063- 1.210	5- 12	Cholesterol Phospholipids	Apo A-I, Apo A-II, Apo C, Apo E
Lp (a)	1.055- 1.085	~30	Cholesterol	Apo B-100, Apo (a)

Table source: https://www.ncbi.nlm.nih.gov/books/NBK305896

Each of the lipoproteins have various responsibilities in the transport of triglycerides and cholesterol around the body:

- The absorption and transport of dietary lipids in the small intestine – known as the exogenous lipoprotein pathway (chylomicrons)
- Transporting lipids from the liver to peripheral tissues – known as the endogenous lipoprotein pathway (VLDL, IDL, LDL, Lp(a))
- Transporting lipids from the peripheral tissues to the liver and intestines – known as the reverse cholesterol transport (HDL)

Before we look at the lipoprotein responsibilities in detail, let's quickly look at apolipoproteins. These are proteins that form part of the membrane of each of the different lipoproteins, and have four major roles:

- Maintaining structural integrity of a lipoprotein
- Ligands for lipoprotein receptors (a ligand is a molecule that bonds with a receptor)
- Formation of lipoproteins
- Activating enzymes that metabolise lipoproteins

There are several different apolipoproteins (six major classes in fact):

- APO-A
    - APO-A1 is associated with HDL
    - APO-A5 is a thought to be a genetic marker leading to raised triglycerides
- APO-B
    - APO-B48 is associated with LDL and chylomicrons formed from food that is consumed
    - APO-B100 is associated with VLDL formed in the liver
- APO-C
    - APO-C2 activates lipoprotein lipase enzyme (you'll learn about this soon)
    - APO-C3 inhibits lipoprotein lipase enzyme and hepatic lipase enzyme

- APO-D
  - APO-D is associated with HDL
- APO-E
  - APO-E is associated with IDL and chylomicron remnants
  - APO-E4 is implicated in atherosclerosis, Alzheimer's disease, and cognitive issues
- APO-H
  - APO-H is also known as glycoprotein I, beta-2 (B2gp1)

OK, now that I've distracted you with apolipoproteins, let's get back to the lipoprotein responsibilities.

Exogenous lipoprotein pathway:

When we eat a meal, large quantities of fatty acids are produced. These are toxic to the body, so they are grouped into triglycerides and cholesterol ester, covered with a layer of phospholipids and apolipoproteins – mainly APO-B48. These now become known as a chylomicron lipoprotein. The chylomicron lipoprotein can travel through the bloodstream with its triglyceride passengers until it meets a lipoprotein lipase enzyme (LPL) in muscle, heart, and adipose tissues. The LPL enzyme releases the fatty acids from the triglycerides, to allow them to be stored in adipose tissues or used as fuel for skeletal or cardiac muscles. The remaining chylomicron is now a chylomicron remnant, headed for the liver.

Endogenous lipoprotein pathway:

Formed similarly to the chylomicron lipoproteins, very low-density lipoproteins (VLDL's) are formed in the liver as triglycerides covered with a layer of phospholipids and apolipoproteins (mainly APO-B100). The newly formed VLDL heads out on a similar journey through the blood stream until its passengers meet a similar fate with the lipoprotein lipase enzyme in the muscle, heart, and adipose tissues, changing the VLDL to an intermediate density lipoprotein (IDL). IDL then sets off again, primarily headed for the liver where it is further metabolised to low density lipoprotein (LDL) by hepatic lipase on the surface of the liver cells, and then accepted via LDL receptors that are waiting for them.

Reverse cholesterol transport

High density lipoproteins (HDL) are formed in the liver and intestines with phospholipids and apolipoproteins APO-A1 and APO-A2, and travel through the bloodstream acquiring cholesterol and phospholipids from cells to form mature HDL. The mature HDL transports its cholesterol passengers directly to the liver itself, or by handing some over to VLDL or LDL on the way.

If that was all a bit too much, here's a simpler analogy. If you're not into analogies, then skip this section...

Think of lipoproteins as buses.

The apolipoproteins on those buses are the bus drivers, allowing the passengers to board, and deciding where the buses are heading.

Cholesterol and triglycerides can't drive, so they're the passengers on the buses.

The road those buses are travelling on is the blood flowing through the veins and arteries.

There are various bus stops that the buses visit, and two bus depots where the buses start/terminate. The main bus depot is the liver and there is a smaller but still significant depot in the intestines. There are bus stops scattered among the muscles, cardiac tissue, and adipose tissue.

At the bus stops and depots, inspectors can be found, ready to assist with the disembarkation of passengers. These inspectors are the lipoprotein lipase enzyme in the muscles, adipose, and cardiac tissues, and the hepatic enzyme in the liver cells.

Got that? OK, strap in, and let's go on a journey...

APO-B48 is the bus driver of the chylomicron bus. This bus starts at the intestine depot, where it picks up its triglyceride passengers and transports them along the road to the various muscle, cardiac, and adipose tissue bus stops where the bus inspectors are waiting to help. Once it's dropped off all its passengers, the remnants of the chylomicron bus heads to the liver depot as a shell of its old self, ready to be recycled/reused when it reaches the liver depot.

APO-B100 is the driver for the VLDL bus which starts its engine in the liver depot where the triglyceride passengers board. The VLDL bus transports them along the road to the same destinations as the chylomicron bus. Once the passengers have been assisted off the bus by the bus inspectors the VLDL bus changes route and becomes an IDL bus, heading back along the road to the liver depot. At the liver depot, another very helpful inspector changes its route again – now it's an LDL bus, and it is directed towards an LDL entry point at the liver depot.

APO-A1 is the bus driver for the HDL bus. This bus is empty as it leaves the liver depot, travelling along the road to the muscles and tissue to pick up cholesterol passengers from any bus stops looking to move on excess passengers. Once full, the HDL bus heads back along the road to the liver depot where the bus driver hands over the passengers ready to be removed from the body. The empty HDL bus turns around and heads back out to the muscles and tissues again. Sometimes, the HDL bus doesn't take the passengers all the way back to the liver and will transfer some of its passengers to the VLDL or LDL buses instead – these passengers take the scenic route to the liver depot or, as my Nan would have said, those passengers get to go all around the houses on their way to the depot.

Did that make things any clearer for you? Possibly not, but if nothing else, now you have a glimpse into how my head works.

References

https://www.ncbi.nlm.nih.gov/books/NBK538139

https://medlineplus.gov/genetics/gene/lcat/

https://www.heart.org/en/health-topics/cholesterol/about-cholesterol

https://academic.oup.com/ehjcimaging/article/20/8/873/5520648

https://www.nhs.uk/conditions/high-cholesterol/

https://www.nhs.uk/conditions/high-cholesterol/how-to-lower-your-cholesterol/

https://pubmed.ncbi.nlm.nih.gov/26055276

https://www.ncbi.nlm.nih.gov/books/NBK305896/

https://www.researchgate.net/figure/Lipoprotein-metabolism-overview-Lipid-distribution-in-the-body-occurs-in-three-different_fig1_357090873

CHAPTER 2: TESTING CARDIOVASCULAR MARKERS

The NHS recommends testing cholesterol if your client is/has:

- Aged 40+ and not had cholesterol levels tested before
- Overweight / raised BMI / high waist measurement (>80cm women, >94cm men)
- Raised blood pressure
- Diagnosed with diabetes
- Family history of raised blood pressure or heart issues

And if other risk factors for heart disease are present:

- No/minimal physical inactivity, or not getting enough exercise
- Previous history of CVD, heart disease, stroke
- Smoking
- Unhealthy eating habits

They also recommend that cholesterol levels should be reviewed every 5 years from the age of 40 onwards, as part of an NHS health check.

Have you ever seen a client in clinic with a private blood test showing a raised LDL in their lipids panel, and not quite known what else should be tested to evaluate the lipids panel appropriately? Simply referring a client back to their doctor with an abnormally raised LDL, together with other risk factors (e.g. smoking, diabetes/pre-diabetes) may cause the doctor to prescribe a statin. This is frustrating when there are further tests that can be done to evaluate the LDL further, and changes to dietary/lifestyle to improve lipid levels.

Having the knowledge to write a well-structured letter to a client's doctor to request a series of blood tests relevant to their symptoms, and then having the confidence to interpret those results, is priceless when it comes to helping clients with their hormonal issues.

Not every client will need tests, but your client will be expecting you as their therapist to decide whether they need them or not.

When writing a letter to a doctor, using medical terms and respectful language can go a long way towards encouraging a doctor to run tests, as it may reassure them that their patient is in safe hands once the results come through.

But as I always say, writing the letter is only step 1.

Interpreting the results and knowing the difference between normal and optimal ranges, and what impact this may have on your client, is the next vital step. As you may have noticed since you graduated, clients presenting in clinic with normal blood results from their doctor do not necessarily have zero symptoms or perfect health.

When you have the confidence to interpret the results, and know what action needs to be taken, your client will no longer find themselves going from doctor to doctor, or therapist to therapist, in their desperate search for answers.

This book will cover selecting the tests, writing the letter, and how to interpret the tests. Let's start with selecting the tests.

Deciding Which Tests to Request

A standard lipids panel markers provided to an individual seeing their doctor usually includes:

- Total cholesterol (TC)
- LDL-cholesterol (LDL)
- HDL-cholesterol (HDL)
- Triglycerides (TG)

It may also include non-HDL cholesterol (non-HDL), TG:HDL ratio, and Total Cholesterol:HDL ratio, but these are easy to calculate if not provided.

A review of blood pressure is often routinely taken at the same time as a lipids panel, especially when it is taken as part of an NHS health check.

Advanced lipids panels are available privately, or through a referral to an NHS lipid clinic, and should include:

- sdLDL
- Lp(a)
- Apolipoprotein A-I
- Apolipoprotein B
- Apolipoprotein B / A-I Ratio
- Apolipoprotein CII
- Apolipoprotein CIII
- Apolipoprotein D
- Apolipoprotein E

To assess risk factors for atherosclerotic cardiovascular disease, glycated haemoglobin (HbA1C) and inflammatory markers may also be tested:

- ESR
- HS-CRP
- HbA1C
- Fasting Glucose
- Fasting Insulin

These markers can be used to calculate HOMA-IR (Homeostatic Model Assessment of Insulin Resistance) and gain an understanding of whether there is likely to be some insulin resistance which may contribute to atherosclerotic cardiovascular disease.

An additional test to consider, particularly in the case or raised total/LDL cholesterol results, would be:

- Coronary Arterial Calcium Scan (CACS)

Considered a minimally invasive method to assess absolute risk of atherosclerotic cardiovascular disease in individuals, a coronary arterial calcium scan (CACS) is a CT scan of the heart that allows for detection and measurement of calcium-rich plaques in the arteries. The only cause of calcium presence in the arteries is atherosclerosis, so its presence is confirmation of the presence of atherosclerotic cardiovascular disease, however there is still a small risk of having atherosclerotic cardiovascular disease even with a score of zero.

This test is currently only available for individuals through a referral to an NHS lipid clinic or privately, and in many cases a scan will only be offered if an individual is presenting with raised blood pressure, raised cholesterol, diabetes, and/or obesity, although it's also recommended for individuals with a strong family history of atherosclerotic cardiovascular disease.

CACS scoring is particularly useful for asymptomatic individuals with raised lipid markers, who are not sure whether statins or other lipid-lowering medications are right for them.

CACS scores range from zero to over 1000, with no maximum range, and scores are used to assess risk of atherosclerotic cardiovascular disease in the next 2-5 years. A CACS score of zero suggests a very low risk of atherosclerotic cardiovascular disease, even in individuals diagnosed with diabetes, raised cholesterol, advanced age, or other risk factors. Higher scores correlate with an increased risk of atherosclerotic cardiovascular disease and should be used to commence dietary and lifestyle changes in the individual.

Coronary artery calcium score	Risk of Atherosclerotic Cardiovascular Event
0	None
0-10	Minimum
11-100	Mild
101-400	Moderate
401-1000	Severe
>1000	Very severe

CACS should be repeated every five years to monitor arterial health. This is especially important in individuals following their CACS score to decide whether statins and other lipid-lowering medications are required.

With the range of tests available through private testing labs, it can be tempting to select all these tests for every single one of your clients. However, this may backfire quickly in the case of NHS referrals, as the doctor may have to refuse the tests simply because they are not available without a lipid clinic referral, or because the client has been tested recently. That same doctor may also tell their patient (your client) that you appear to be wasting their time and NHS money and services. This will not boost your reputation as a nutritional therapist at all.

Even for a basic lipids panel, which is widely available and routinely tested, you will also need to consider if the client has been tested for it in the past 5 years. If they have, but you still feel it should be retested, then you will need to be able to justify the reason for requesting a retest. A lot can change in 5 years, particularly with diet and lifestyle changes, such as when working with a nutritional therapist, and this is where private testing can be useful.

To avoid the "kid in a sweet shop" feeling when looking at blood tests that are available, and to avoid wasting your client's time, money, and blood, I use my tried and tested method to narrow down which bloods to request. Starting with a list of every test available, remove any that are:

- Not relevant
- Unjustifiable based on my client's symptoms

If requesting tests through the client's doctor, I also remove any that are:

- Not available without referral to lipid clinic (see page 33)
- Have been tested within past 12 months (HbA1C) or past 5 years (lipids panel) without justifiable reason for retesting

Over the years, I have refined this method and have created my Cardiovascular Blood Testing Matrix. This matrix includes a list of cardiovascular symptoms or risk criteria that a client may have, matched up to a list of relevant cardiovascular-related blood tests that I might then request.

To ensure that you don't fall into the trap of requesting too many blood tests, or not testing the right markers, I will share my Cardiovascular Blood Testing Matrix with you on the following pages. When used in conjunction with a client consultation, the matrix may help you to select the right tests for determining your client's cardiovascular status.

References

https://www.ultalabtests.com/testing/categories/heart-and-cardiovascular/cholesterol?page=2

https://www.nhs.uk/conditions/high-cholesterol/getting-tested/

https://www.heartuk.org.uk/low-cholesterol-foods/looking-after-your-weight

https://www.nhs.uk/conditions/statins/

https://pubmed.ncbi.nlm.nih.gov/22079127/

https://www.ncbi.nlm.nih.gov/pmc/articles/PMC3384065/

https://patient.info/doctor/coronary-artery-calcium-score

https://www.houstonmethodist.org/blog/articles/2021/oct/calcium-score-what-s-a-cac-test-do-i-need-one/

Cardiovascular Blood Testing Matrix

	Basic Lipids Panel	Advanced Lipids Profile	HbA1C	C-Peptide	Fasting Insulin	Fasting Glucose	HS-CRP	ESR	Coronary Arterial Calcium
Aged 40+ and not aware of cholesterol levels	X		X				X	X	
Previous history of dyslipidaemia	X	X	X	X	X	X	X	X	X
Raised blood pressure	X		X				X	X	
Diagnosed with diabetes Types 1, 1.5 (LADA), or 2	X	X	X	X	X	X	X	X	
Poor eating habits	X		X	X	X	X	X	X	
Sedentary lifestyle	X		X		X	X	X	X	
Increased waist measurement	X		X	X	X	X	X	X	
Family history of dyslipidaemia	X		X				X	X	X
Family history of raised blood pressure	X		X				X	X	
Family history of cardiovascular disease	X	X	X	X	X	X	X	X	X
Clubbed fingers	X		X				X	X	
Ear lobe creasing (Frank's sign)	X		X				X	X	
Xanthomata presence	X	X	X	X	X	X	X	X	
Chronic Kidney Disease / Nephrotic Kidneys	X	X	X	X	X	X	X	X	X

CHAPTER 3: CARDIOVASCULAR RED FLAGS

In addition to the red flags mentioned in my previous books, these red flags relate to cardiovascular health and will require referral back to the client's doctor for further investigation:

Symptoms of Coronary Heart Disease:

- Chest pain
- Shortness of breath
- Generalised pain in the body
- Feeling faint
- Nausea

Symptoms of High Blood Pressure:

High blood pressure rarely has noticeable symptoms, although the following can be symptoms of high blood pressure:

- Blurred vision
- Nosebleeds
- Shortness of breath
- Chest pain
- Dizziness
- Headaches

Symptoms of congestive heart failure:

- Oedema of ankles/legs which may be better in the mornings, but gradually get worse later in the day
- Shortness of breath after activities
- Shortness of breath when laying down
- Waking up with shortness of breath in the night
- Feeling tired all the time
- Unable to exercise due to fatigue
- Feeling lightheaded, and fainting

Symptoms of angina:

- Tight, dull, or heavy chest pain
- Sharp, stabbing chest pain
- Chest pain that spreads to arms, neck, jaw, or back
- Chest pain that is triggered by physical exertion and/or stressful situations
- Chest pain that stops when resting
- Shortness of breath

Symptoms of a stroke:

The mnemonic FAST (face – arms – speech – time) can be used to identify the main symptoms of a stroke.

- Face – drooping on one side, unable to smile, mouth/eye drooping
- Arms – weakness or numbness in one arm – they may be unable to lift both arms and keep them raised

- Speech – slurring, garbled, unable to speak despite appearing conscious, unable to understand what you are saying to them
- Time – call 999 immediately if you notice any of these signs or symptoms.

The symptoms of a stroke may also include:

- Paralysis of one side of the body
- Sudden loss of vision
- Sudden onset of blurred vision
- Sudden onset of double vision
- Vertigo
- Vomiting
- Dizziness
- Confusion
- Unable to understand what you are saying to them
- Unable to balance or poor coordination
- Dysphagia

Symptoms of a TIA:

The symptoms of a transient ischaemic attack (TIA) may be identical to those of a stroke but lasting only a few minutes or hours.

Symptoms of Peripheral Arterial Disease

- Intermittent claudication (painful ache in legs when walking that eases with rest)
- Alopecia of legs and feet

- Numbness or weakness in legs
- Brittle and slow growing toenails
- Ulcers on the feet and legs that do not heal
- Paler or blue-toned skin on legs
- Skin becoming shinier
- Erectile dysfunction in men
- Sarcopenia (wasting of muscles) in legs

Symptoms of Aortic Disease

Aortic aneurysms can occur anywhere in the aorta, and include abdominal aortic aneurysms (AAA), and thoracic aortic aneurysms (TAA).

Individuals with AAA may present with:

- A pulsing sensation in the abdomen
- Persistent abdominal pain
- Persistent lower back pain

Individuals with TAA may present with:

- Deep, aching, throbbing chest pain
- Back pain
- Coughing or shortness of breath
- Hoarseness
- Dysphagia (trouble swallowing)
- Odynophagia (painful swallowing)

A burst AAA or TAA requires urgent medical attention. Call 999 if your client is reporting:

- Severe pain
- Dizziness and fainting
- Sweaty, pale, and clammy skin
- Tachycardia
- Shortness of breath

Symptoms of a Heart Attack

- Persistent chest pain
  - Pressure in the chest
  - Heaviness in the chest
  - Tightness in the chest
  - Squeezing across the chest
- Pain that spreads from chest to arms (left or both), jaw, neck, back, abdomen
- Dizziness
- Sweating
- Shortness of breath
- Nausea or vomiting
- Coughing or wheezing
- Overwhelming feeling of anxiety
- Unconsciousness
- Seizures or fitting
- Difficulty breathing
- Tachycardia
- Blue or pale tingling of knees, hands, lips

- Coughing up blood

Symptoms of a Cardiac Arrest:

Call 999 and start chest compressions if your client suddenly presents with:

- Not breathing
- Not moving
- No pulse
- Not responding to stimulation e.g. being touched, or spoken to

Other Symptoms:

- Chronic pancreatitis (may be linked with raised triglycerides)
- Palpitations
- Irregular heartbeat
- Frank's Sign (ear lobe creases) ← a symptom to prompt further testing, rather than a red flag
- Clubbing of fingertips ← a symptom to prompt further testing, rather than a red flag
- Tendon Xanthomata
  - o Build-up of cholesterol deep within tendons or ligaments
  - o Presents on fingers, feet, and Achilles tendon
  - o Associated with raised LDL and hypercholesterolaemia
- Tuberous Xanthomata

- o Red/yellow papules and nodules 0.5-2.5cm diameter
- o Presents on knees, elbows, heels, and buttocks
- o Associated with raised LDL and hypercholesterolaemia
- Eruptive Xanthomata
    - o Small, yellow, tender, pruritic lesions, and papules
    - o Presents anywhere on body, except on the face
    - o Associated with hypertriglyceridaemia and/or type 2 diabetes
- Plane Xanthomata
    - o Multiple yellow/orange elevated papules and plaques
    - o Presents anywhere on the body
    - o Associated with lipid abnormalities
- Palmar Xanthomata
    - o Multiple yellow/orange raised papules and plaques
    - o Presents on creases of palm of the hand
    - o Associated with lipid abnormalities
- Xanthelasmata
    - o Symmetrical lesions on eyelid or near inner eye
    - o Associated with raised LDL
- Corneal Arcus

- White, blue, or grey arc or ring appearing around cornea of eye
- Associated with aging, hypertriglyceridaemia, excess alcohol

-

If in doubt, always refer your client to their doctor for further investigations.

References

https://www.nhs.uk/conditions/cardiovascular-disease/

https://www.nhs.uk/conditions/heart-failure/symptoms/

https://www.nhs.uk/conditions/angina/symptoms/

https://www.nhs.uk/conditions/stroke/symptoms/

https://www.nhs.uk/conditions/transient-ischaemic-attack-tia/symptoms/

https://www.nhs.uk/conditions/peripheral-arterial-disease-pad/

https://www.nhs.uk/conditions/coronary-heart-disease/

https://www.nhs.uk/conditions/abdominal-aortic-aneurysm/

https://stanfordhealthcare.org/medical-conditions/blood-heart-circulation/thoracic-aortic-aneurysm/symptoms.html

https://www.nhs.uk/conditions/heart-attack/symptoms/

https://www.nhs.uk/conditions/heart-attack/symptoms/

https://www.nhsinform.scot/illnesses-and-conditions/heart-and-blood-vessels/conditions/heart-attack

https://www.bhf.org.uk/informationsupport/conditions/familial-hypercholesterolaemia

https://www.pcds.org.uk/clinical-guidance/xanthomata

CHAPTER 4: WRITING TO THE CLIENT'S DOCTOR

As already mentioned in my previous books, the best service you can offer to your client as their therapist, is to write a letter for their doctor.

Writing to doctors, whether NHS or private, can be overwhelming. The imposter syndrome kicks in, and we can't imagine a doctor wanting to listen to our recommendations for testing. But remember – you are likely to have spent significantly more time with your client than they will have spent with their doctor. They may have mentioned symptoms or lifestyle habits that ring alarm bells for cardiovascular health, but that would not have been raised during a 7-minute consultation with their doctor due to lack of time.

Although your client has come to see you, they are still their doctor's patient, and I would recommend being clear on this in the letter. You are not trying to take them away from their doctor, and this isn't an "us versus them" situation. You are providing a complementary therapy, and you need to work with their doctor to provide the level of support that your client is expecting. As such, the letter will need to convey this message to the doctor in a clear and succinct manner.

The letter will need to be formally structured and should include:

1. Your clinic name, address, and logo
2. The date of the letter
3. The doctor surgery name and address (if known)
4. A suitable opening to the letter
    a. Dear Dr. *name* (if known)
    b. Dear Sir/Madam
5. Patient identifying details
    a. Patient name
    b. Patient DOB
    c. Patient home address
6. Introduction of yourself to the client's doctor, with details of your registrations or qualifications where relevant
7. An outline of their patient's current symptoms, taken from the test matrix
8. The reasons for your concerns, or any research/relevant guidelines to justify testing
9. The list of tests you would like them to have done, taken from the test matrix
10. A suitable sign-off to the letter
    a. Yours sincerely (if addressed Dear Dr. *name*)
    b. Your faithfully (if addressed Dear Sir/Madam)

That's a lot of information to fit into one letter, but I will now take you through how you can fit all of that into one letter without it going on for pages and pages.

Formatting the Letter

Ensuring your letter includes items 1-5 from the list is self-explanatory.

For example:

Sunrise Nutrition Clinic
14 Upmile Lane
London
EC2N 4DS
23rd March 2023

Snowy Medical Centre
Snow Drive
RF2 1DF

Dear Sir/Madam (or Dear Dr. Thray etc.)

Re: Ms. Anastasia Smith, DOB: 12/04/1980, Address: 45 Mill Road, RF2 1DD

To introduce yourself, start with "I am a *therapist role including registrations etc.* and met your patient, *client name*, in my clinic on the *date in clinic* presenting with *list of symptoms relevant to the tests you are requesting*"

For example:

I am a registered nutritional therapist (BANT, CNHC) and met your patient, Ms. Smith, in my clinic on the 10th ^{of} March 2023 presenting with....

For the symptoms, group together any symptoms that you believe may be related to one underlying cause/trigger and always lead with any red flags, followed by "together with...." And the list of other symptoms.

Where relevant, you should explain your reasons for wishing to get the client tested such as red flags, and/or referring to any relevant guidelines when describing your client's symptoms. Remember that doctors may be restricted in the tests they can offer, so using these guidelines when describing symptoms may encourage/enable to doctor to provide the relevant tests.

Including copies of relevant research that supports your requests may help but do remember that doctors may not have the time to read through large research studies during a 7-minute appointment.

For example:

...presenting with shortness of breath, raised blood pressure, and a family history of hyperlipidaemia and cardiovascular disease, together with a waist measurement of 100cm. I would very much appreciate your assistance with running the following tests to rule

out any such underlying functional causes of their
symptoms...

NOTE: At no point should you lie about the symptoms
that your client has. If you are not able to justify
requesting additional tests that you feel your client needs,
you will need to consider testing privately.

If the client has done any relevant private tests or has
previous test results that are relevant to your requests in
this letter, mention these at this point too, and attach
them to the letter where relevant.

For example:

I note that Ms. Smith had her lipids profile tested in 2012
and her total cholesterol was borderline raised at
5mmol/L, but there have been no further tests since.

To ensure the right tests are offered, it would be a good
idea to list them in the letter at this point.

For example:

To provide Ms. Smith with a suitable nutrition plan, I
would very much appreciate your assistance with running
the following tests to review her current cholesterol
markers and rule out any such underlying functional
causes of her symptoms:

- Lipids profile
- HbA1C

Add a sign-off to the letter, appropriate to the opening used at the start of the letter.

For example:

Dear Sir/Madam,

Content of the letter requesting tests

Yours faithfully,

Kate Knowler

Or

Dear Dr. Thray,

Content of the letter requesting tests

Yours sincerely,

Kate Knowler

In the footer section of your letter you can include any qualifications, registrations, and governing bodies.

Once typed, save the file according to your regional data protection policies, and arrange for a copy to be sent to the client's doctor either by email, post, or given to the client to hand-deliver themselves.

I personally prefer to email the letter directly to the doctor's surgery, with permission from the client (obtained as part of their case history) and email a copy to the client. I advise the client to book an appointment with their doctor to discuss the letter. This way, the doctor has a copy of my requests showing my analysis, even if the client chooses not to go to the doctor to get tests done. This is especially important in cases that involve red flags.

Language to use in referral letters

Doctors use a different language from their patients and as the mediator, we need to be able to discuss in normal everyday terms with our clients but use medical terms when writing to the doctor.

Using medical terms will also earn some respect with the doctor and provide them with a level of reassurance that you know what you are talking about.

Here are some examples to use when discussing cardiovascular symptoms and blood tests. Blood Labs 1 and 2 also include other markers related to fatigue and sex hormones respectively.

- Breathless or shortness of breath – dyspnoea
- Tired all the time – fatigue despite adequate sleep
- Raised cholesterol levels – dyslipidaemia
- Raised triglycerides – hypertriglyceridaemia
- Dizziness – presyncope

- Fainting – syncope
- Difficulty swallowing – dysphagia
- Painful swallowing – odynophagia

Testing Privately

If the doctor has refused to test or is likely to refuse to provide all the tests that you would like to request, or your client has expressed a preference for choosing a private testing facility rather than their doctor (perhaps due to time constraints, or because they are looking for an independent second opinion), then you have several choices.

Private testing laboratories are available with options such as home finger-prick tests or dried blood spot tests, home/work nurse phlebotomy visits to draw the blood, or private phlebotomy appointments in clinics or hospitals.

Phlebotomy is the act of drawing blood from a patient's veins. Home finger-prick and dried blood spot tests do not require phlebotomy as they draw blood from the fingertips rather than a vein, and they are also more limited on the markers available to test due to the smaller sample size.

If your client is doing a finger-prick test, here are some tips for improving the blood supply to the finger prior to using the lancet to prick the finger:

- Ensure they are well hydrated – this should be assessed over the previous 24 hours, not just a glass of water prior to using the lancet
- Prepare the test tube for blood collection (open it, place it somewhere safe)
- Fill the kitchen sink with hot water – a little hotter than usual but not hot enough to burn the hands
- Soak the hands for 5 minutes – they can even do the washing up during this time!
- After 5 minutes in the warm water, remove the hands from the water and dry them with a clean towel or disposable paper towel
- Do 10 seconds of exercise involving moving their arms e.g. star jumps, swinging the arms around etc.
- Wipe the fingertip with an alcohol wipe included in the test kit, and allow the alcohol to evaporate from the finger
- Prick the finger with the lancet
- Wipe away the first spot of blood, and then proceed with collecting the blood sample
- If they find that blood flow slows while taking the sample, get them to repeat the above process, pricking on a different finger.

Finger-prick testing is not suitable for everybody. If your client is struggling to obtain a sample, recommend that they call the blood test lab to discuss alternative phlebotomy options.

If your client is young, has poor circulation, is prone to being squeamish, has an aversion to blood, or is in any way unsure about finger-prick testing, then I would recommend choosing an alternative phlebotomy option rather than a finger-prick test. This prevents the risk of wasting your clients' time/energy/fingertips attempting to squeeze out a few drops of blood from their finger.

Private labs that I have used in the UK include Blue Horizon Medicals, Healthpath Pro, Thriva, Medichecks, and Randox, but there are others.

Things to check when choosing a private laboratory, aside from the price of the test and the markers being tested, include:

- Is the cost of phlebotomy included
- If not, do they have a list of available phlebotomists that you can approach
- After-care support e.g. doctor writeup of the results
- Support for finger-prick tests if the client has any issues

If your client does test privately, it's worth making them aware that you will be obliged to advise their doctor of any abnormal results in their private tests, and that their doctor may then choose to repeat the tests.

To Fast or Not to Fast Before Testing

Fasting is recommended when testing a basic or advanced lipid profile, glucose levels, and insulin levels, but this may not be communicated to your client by their doctor when the tests are requested as the NHS guidelines for fasting vary and testing unfasted is gaining in popularity.

As an experiment for writing this book, I did a fasted lipids profile with Randox Laboratories, followed by 3 hours of eating nothing but carbohydrates and sugar (for the record, this was half a packet of Tesco gluten free shortbread, half a sharing bag of sour Haribo sweets, 250ml of apple juice, a handful of grapes and blueberries, and a few sips of water) and then repeating the same blood test panel.

The results showed that my fasted triglycerides went from 0.46mmol/L to 0.79mmol/L after my sugar feast. I would consider myself to have good control of my blood sugar levels, and eating such a large amount of sugar and carbohydrates is unusual for me. For a client who may eat similar foods on a daily basis the effect may well be less significant. Other noticeable differences for my results after the sugar binge were a decrease in my total cholesterol and LDL levels, and a raise in HDL levels.

My blood results:

	FASTED	NON-FASTED
Total Cholesterol	3.95mmol/L	3.89mmol/L
LDL Cholesterol	2.06mmol/L	1.95mmol/L
HDL Cholesterol	1.37mmol/L	1.41mmol/L
Total:HDL ratio	2.88	2.76
Triglycerides	0.46mmol/L	0.79mmol/L

These patterns of changes may not be the same for every client, and I would have to do more experiments to know for sure, but my recommendation would be that fasted lipid panels are more accurate, and you should explain to your client what this involves:

- No food after midnight the night before testing
- No drinks after midnight the night before testing
- Only water can and should be consumed prior to the test (this is important to ensure the blood draw is successful)

I would also recommend avoiding supplements for 5 days prior to testing, as a precaution.

Never assume that every client will understand what needs to be avoided for a successful fasted blood test. I have had several clients attend for a fasted blood test, holding everything from takeaway coffees to boxes of fruit and cartons of fruit juice, or clients that have fasted without drinking any water so that they are so dehydrated I'm unable to draw blood from them.

CHAPTER 5: BASIC LIPIDS PROFILE

The basic lipids profile should be available from a client's doctor, and includes some or all of the following:

- Total Cholesterol
- LDL
- HDL
- Non-HDL
- Triglycerides
- Triglycerides:HDL ratio
- Total Cholesterol:HDL ratio

Total Cholesterol

Total Cholesterol is the sum of all the lipoproteins transporting cholesterol and triglycerides in your blood – HDL, LDL, and VLDL. Note that Lp(a) and IDL are not included in the sum, as these are considered to be part of LDL.

In this way, and quite confusingly, Total Cholesterol is not a measure of actual cholesterol in the blood but a measure of all the lipoproteins transporting the cholesterol and triglycerides.

If your client has an NHS lipids panel blood test, they should receive their Total Cholesterol results with or without the other lipids markers. If Total Cholesterol has not been provided, you can estimate it using the following formula:

$$HDL + LDL + (TG \times 0.2) = \text{Total Cholesterol}$$

Raised Total Cholesterol

If Total Cholesterol is raised above the reference range, it's important to investigate the underlying cause – looking at LDL, HDL, and triglyceride levels (and other markers if you have them) and working to address imbalances appropriately.

For example:

- Raised total cholesterol with raised triglycerides should lead you to address diet, insulin resistance, and blood sugar balance.
- Raised total cholesterol with raised LDL should lead you to assess for sdLDL and address the dietary intake of carbohydrates / saturated fats as appropriate.
- Raised total cholesterol with raised HDL should lead you to assess diet, medications (e.g. oral contraceptives, HRT, anti-convulsant medications), genetics, menopause, hypothyroidism, infections, inflammation e.g. rheumatoid arthritis.

Pregnancy may also influence cholesterol levels and clients should wait 6 weeks after giving birth before retesting their cholesterol levels.

Decreased Total Cholesterol

Total Cholesterol below the optimal range may be associated with:

- Increased risk of haemorrhagic stroke e.g. primary intracerebral haemorrhage
- Depression & anxiety
- Low vitamin D
- Low sex hormones
- Low steroid hormones
- Poor bile production

- Possible increased risk of cancer
- Preterm birth and low birth weight if cholesterol is low during pregnancy

Total Cholesterol Reference Range

Total Cholesterol is measured in millimoles per litre (mmol/L)

- Normal Range: 4.1 - 5mmol/L

References

https://www.healthline.com/health/cholesterol-can-it-be-too-low

https://corporate.dukehealth.org/news/women-low-cholesterol-may-be-risk-depression-and-anxiety

https://www.acc.org/about-acc/press-releases/2012/03/25/15/15/ldl_cancer

https://onlinelibrary.wiley.com/doi/abs/10.1002/lite.201000070

https://pubmed.ncbi.nlm.nih.gov/10367605/

https://journals.lww.com/annalsofian/Fulltext/2012/15010/Low_cholesterol_as_a_risk_factor_for_primary.6.aspx

Low Density Lipoprotein – LDL

Often considered to be the "lousy" or "bad" cholesterol, raised LDL is the trigger for prescribing statins. However, LDL is now known to be formed of 7 subtypes:

- Types 1-2 considered non-pathogenic, large buoyant LDL, with a diameter ≥ 25.5nm
- Types 3-7 considered pathogenic, small dense LDL, with a diameter <25.5nm

If you're looking for an analogy here, consider the large buoyant LDL as large fluffy clouds or beach balls, bouncing along the arteries doing no damage, and the small dense LDL as small, hard bullets, pushing and shoving their way through the arteries and looking to cause a problem.

Large buoyant LDL (lbLDL) subtypes are considered to bring less atherosclerotic cardiovascular disease risk than small dense LDL (sdLDL) subtypes. Long term dietary consumption of saturated fat appears to raise lbLDL levels, while long term dietary consumption of carbohydrates appears to raise sdLDL

Used alone, LDL is no longer considered a reliable marker of cardiovascular risk, and it is important to test or estimate the LDL subtypes as well as look at non-HDL and the ratios.

Nordic Labs offer the LDL Liposcan test for looking at the LDL subtype breakdown – this test requires phlebotomy and centrifuging but produces a very comprehensive breakdown of the LDL subtypes.

A link to a spreadsheet for calculating sdLDL is discussed in the sdLDL section of this chapter.

When reported in test results, LDL is either calculated or directly measured.

The three calculation methods are the Friedewald equation, the Martin/Hopkins equation, and the NIH equation.

The Friedewald equation estimates LDL as:

$$\text{Total Cholesterol} - \text{HDL} - (\text{TG} \div 5) = \text{LDL}$$

The Martin/Hopkins equation estimates LDL using an adjustable factor based on triglyceride:VLDL ratio:

$$\text{Total Cholesterol} - \text{HDL} - (\text{TG} \div \text{adjustable factor})$$

The National Institutes of Health (NIH) equation estimates LDL as:

$$(\text{Total Cholesterol} \div 0.948) - (\text{HDL} \div 0.971) - (\,(\text{TG} \div 8.56)$$
$$+ ((\text{TG} \times \text{Non-HDL}) \div 2140) - (\text{TG}^2 \div 16100)\,) - 9.44$$

For clients with hypertriglyceridaemia, the NIH equation is the most reliable for calculating LDL although if triglycerides are too raised (over 9mmol/L, e.g. with a metabolic disease that affects lipid and triglyceride levels) a direct LDL test would be required.

Raised LDL

LDL above the optimal range may be associated with:

- Dietary intake of saturated fats, carbohydrates, sugars
- Smoking
- Excess alcohol intake
- Lack of exercise
- Genetic pre-disposition e.g. familial hypercholesterolaemia

If your client has raised LDL, particularly if they also have decreased HDL, you should consider evaluating sdLDL and a coronary arterial calcium scan (CACS).

Decreased LDL

LDL below the optimal range may be associated with:

- Cholesterol lowering medications e.g. Statins
- Malnourishment e.g. poor intake of nutrients or inability to absorb nutrients from diet
- Hyperthyroidism
- Chronic infections e.g. hepatitis C
- Chronic inflammation
- Blood cancers
- Genetic predisposition e.g. familial hypobetalipoproteinaemia, chylomicron retention disease, abetalipoproteinaemia

LDL Reference Range

LDL is measured in millimoles per litre (mmol/L)

- Normal Range: 1.2-3mmol/L

References:

https://www.healthline.com/health/cholesterol-can-it-be-too-low

https://www.sciencedirect.com/science/article/abs/pii/S0009912015000338

https://academic.oup.com/jalm/article/6/5/1384/6328868

https://www.ncbi.nlm.nih.gov/books/NBK542294/

https://www.zora.uzh.ch/id/eprint/73838/2/Regulation_of_low-density_lipoportein-PhG.pdf

https://journals.sagepub.com/doi/10.1258/acb.2010.010185

https://www.bmj.com/content/347/bmj.f6340/rr/669222

https://pubmed.ncbi.nlm.nih.gov/14505481/

https://pubmed.ncbi.nlm.nih.gov/23627975/

https://stanfordlab.com/articles/equation-for-low-density-lipoprotein-cholesterol-calculation.html

High Density Lipoprotein – HDL

HDL is often considered to be the "happy" or "healthy" cholesterol, as it is thought to protect heart and blood vessels from disease in the following ways:

- Collects cholesterol from blood vessels and other tissues and transports to the liver for elimination in the reverse cholesterol transport
- Anti-inflammatory – HDL appears to inhibit recruitment of monocytes into the arterial walls by inhibiting endothelial cell adhesion molecules
- Antioxidant – Apolipoproteins (remember our bus drivers in chapter 1?) APO-A1 and APO-A2 protect LDL cholesterol from oxidation

Lower HDL increases the risk of atherosclerotic cardiovascular disease.

HDL carries approximately one quarter of the cholesterol in the bloodstream at any one time. The remaining three quarters of the cholesterol is found in the other lipoproteins e.g. LDL, VLDL, IDL.

Raised HDL

Increased levels of HDL may be associated with:

- Overexercising
- Dietary intake of saturated fats
- Excess alcohol intake
- Medications: phenytoin, insulin, oestrogen

To improve HDL levels, review the suggestions made in Chapter 10: Modifiable Diet and Lifestyle Risk Factors.

Decreased HDL

Low levels of HDL may be associated with:

- Smoking – changes structure of APO-A1
- Insulin resistance
- Type 2 diabetes
- Excess abdominal adipose tissue
- Medicines: Beta blockers, thiazide diuretics, oral contraceptives, anabolic steroids
- Genetic predisposition e.g. Tangier disease, APO-A1 deficiency, familial combined hyperlipidaemia (FCH)

Note: a client's HDL levels may lower temporarily when they are, or have been, unwell. HDL may also be lower after a heart attack or following a stressful incident such as surgery or heart attack. It is recommended to wait 6 weeks after illness before testing cholesterol levels.

With regards to medications, statins are used to lower LDL levels, but do not change HDL levels; fibrates are used to lower triglycerides and may have a small effect on HDL levels; Ezetimibe and PCSK9 monoclonal antibodies e.g. Alirocumab and Evolocumab, may raise HDL levels.

HDL Reference Range

HDL is measured in millimoles per litre (mmol/L)

- Normal Male Range: 1-2.3mmol/L
- Normal Female Range: 1.2-2.3mmol/L

HDL benefits peak at 1.4mmol/L. Levels over 1.4mmol/L appear to be of no benefit, and at levels of >2.3mmol/L, the HDL acts more like LDL cholesterol, increasing risk of heart attack or stroke, particularly during perimenopause and post-menopause.

References:

https://labtestsonline.org.uk/tests/hdl-cholesterol-test

https://www.ncbi.nlm.nih.gov/pmc/articles/PMC7470150/

https://www.health.harvard.edu/heart-health/hdl-cholesterol-how-much-is-enough

ps://www.urmc.rochester.edu/encyclopedia/content.aspx?ContentTypeID=167&ContentID=lipid_panel_hdl_ratio

https://www.heartuk.org.uk/genetic-conditions/high-hdl-cholesterol

https://www.heartuk.org.uk/cholesterol/hdl-cholesterol

https://www.ncbi.nlm.nih.gov/pmc/articles/PMC4607861/

https://www.ncbi.nlm.nih.gov/pmc/articles/PMC5597817

https://www.ahajournals.org/doi/10.1161/01.RES.0000146094.59640.13?url_ver=Z39.88-2003&rfr_id=ori:rid:crossref.org&rfr_dat=cr_pub%20%200pubmed

https://www.ahajournals.org/doi/10.1161/CIRCULATIONAHA.120.050808

https://www.ahajournals.org/doi/10.1161/CIRCULATIONAHA.120.050808

https://gpnotebook.com/en-ie/simplepage.cfm?ID=x20030612231634840010

Non-High Density Lipoprotein – Non-HDL

Non-HDL is a calculated value, representing any lipoproteins that are not HDL within the Total Cholesterol value – e.g. LDL, VLDL, IDL, and chylomicrons, all of which have the apolipoprotein APO-B in common.

The formula to calculate non-HDL is:

Total Cholesterol – HDL = Non-HDL

Non-HDL is a strong predictor of atherogenic cardiovascular disease than LDL alone and correlates with APO-B measurement except in clients with dyslipoproteinaemias (disorders of lipid levels, lipoprotein structure, or abnormal lipoprotein composition/density).

Raised Non-HDL

A raised non-HDL may be associated with an increased risk of atherosclerotic cardiovascular disease, and risk factors of raised LDL and decreased HDL should be considered.

Decreased Non-HDL

A decreased non-HDL is considered optimal, and no low threshold has been set.

Non-HDL Reference Range

Non-HDL is measured in millimoles per litre (mmol/L)

- Normal Range: <4mmol/L

References

https://www.heartuk.org.uk/cholesterol/understanding-your-cholesterol-test-results-

https://www.health.harvard.edu/heart-health/what-is-non-hdl-cholesterol

Triglycerides – TG

This is a measure of all the triglycerides found in the VLDL and chylomicrons in the bloodstream.

Triglycerides are compounds, or esters, of glycerol together with three chains of fatty acids. They are the main source of fuel for muscles, and essential for health.

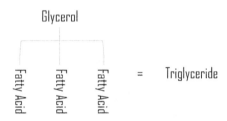

Exogenous triglycerides will raise in the blood after eating a meal, as sugars and fats from the meal are transported by chylomicrons from the intestines to the peripheral tissues and the liver for storage/recirculation.

Endogenous triglycerides are formed in the liver and carried by VLDL, also formed in the liver, to the peripheral tissues for use as a cellular energy source.

Fasting is recommended when testing triglycerides, and this used to be the standard recommendation, although some studies show that readings after a meal are useful, so NHS guidelines vary and testing unfasted is gaining popularity. Always check with your client whether their lipids profile was fasted or not.

Raised Triglycerides

An increased level of triglycerides may be associated with:

- Primary Causes:
    - Familial hypertriglyceridaemia
    - Familial combined hyperlipidaemia (FCH)
    - Type 3 hyperlipidaemia
    - Familial chylomicronaemia syndrome
    - LPL enzyme deficiency
- Secondary Causes:
    - Insulin resistance, uncontrolled DM2
    - Diet high in saturated fats and added sugars
    - Alcohol
    - Sedentary lifestyle
    - Kidney disease
    - NAFLD
    - Gout
    - Pregnancy
    - Hypothyroidism
    - Medications – e.g. some diuretics, steroids, oral oestrogen, retinoids, retrovirals

Hypertriglyceridaemia may cause pancreatitis and may be linked with poor liver and/or biliary function, or poor fat metabolism.

Decreased Triglycerides

Low levels of triglycerides may be associated with:

- Poor release of fatty acids
- Endocrine hyperfunction
- Immune problem
- Low dietary intake

Triglycerides Reference Range

Triglycerides are measured in millimoles per litre (mmol/L)

- Fasting Triglycerides Normal Range: <1.7mmol/L
- Non-Fasting Triglycerides Normal Range: <2.3mmol/L

References:

https://pubmed.ncbi.nlm.nih.gov/20699090/

https://www.heartuk.org.uk/cholesterol/triglycerides

https://www.journal-advocate.com/2012/02/27/the-importance-of-triglyceridehdl-ratio

https://labtestsonline.org.uk/tests/triglycerides

https://www.nhs.uk/conditions/high-cholesterol/getting-tested

https://pubmed.ncbi.nlm.nih.gov/16860278

Triglycerides:HDL ratio – TG:HDL

A high level of triglycerides and low level of HDL is associated with conditions such as insulin resistance, type 2 diabetes, and metabolic syndrome. Indeed, increased TG:HDL ratio is considered one of the diagnostic criteria for metabolic syndrome (along with being overweight and/or excess adipose tissue around the waist, blood pressure over 140/99mmHg, and insulin resistance or inability to control blood sugar levels).

TG:HDL is also considered a strong predictor of heart disease – more so than high cholesterol or raised TC:HDL ratio.

You must convert both triglycerides and HDL into mg/dL (use unitslab.com to do this) and then the formula used to calculate the TG:HDL ratio is:

$$TG \div HDL = TG{:}HDL \text{ ratio}$$

A smaller ratio is achieved with one or both of low triglycerides and raised HDL.

Raised TG:HDL Ratio

An increased TG:HDL ratio would suggest that there is a high level of triglycerides and/or a low level of HDL and is associated with an increased risk of heart disease. To improve the TG:HDL ratio, look at risk factors for raised triglycerides and decreased HDL, and work on stabilising blood pressure levels.

In Chapter 10: Modifiable Diet and Lifestyle Risk Factors, there are suggestions for ways to improve both triglycerides and HDL, which would support improving the TG:HDL ratio.

Decreased TG:HDL Ratio

A lower TG:HDL ratio is associated with a decreased risk of heart disease.

TG:HDL Reference Range

As TG:HDL is a ratio, there are no units.

- Optimal Range: <1.1
- Normal Range: 2-3
- Significant risk of heart attack and stroke: >3

References:

https://www.omnicalculator.com/health/cholesterol-ratio

https://www.nhs.uk/conditions/metabolic-syndrome/

https://www.ncbi.nlm.nih.gov/pmc/articles/PMC6992727

https://pubmed.ncbi.nlm.nih.gov/22565137/

https://www.jstage.jst.go.jp/article/jat/10/3/10_3_186/_pdf/-char/en

https://thebloodcode.com/know-your-tghdl-ratio-triglyceride-hdl-cholesterol/

https://jamanetwork.com/journals/jamainternalmedicine/fullarticle/647239

https://www.ncbi.nlm.nih.gov/pmc/articles/PMC6516523/

https://www.journal-advocate.com/2012/02/27/the-importance-of-triglyceridehdl-ratio

Total Cholesterol:HDL Ratio – TC:HDL

The TC:HDL ratio explores the level of HDL in the blood, compared to the Total Cholesterol levels, and is used alongside the other lipid panel markers to assess atherosclerotic cardiovascular risk.

The formula used to calculate TC:HDL ratio is:

$$\text{Total Cholesterol} \div \text{HDL} = \text{TC:HDL Ratio}$$

Raised TC:HDL Ratio

An increased ratio would indicate that the levels of HDL are not sufficient to provide cardiovascular protection.

To improve the TC:HDL ratio, the suggestions made in Chapter 10: Modifiable Diet and Lifestyle Risk Factors should be followed.

Decreased TC:HDL Ratio

A lower ratio results in a lower risk due to a higher level of HDL levels as a proportion of total cholesterol, providing a protective effect. One 2019 study found women with a TC:HDL ratio of >4 had a significant increase in likelihood of a heart attack.

TC:HDL Reference Range

As TC:HDL is a ratio, there are no units.

- Normal Range: <6
- Optimal Range: ≤ 3.5

References

https://www.medicalnewstoday.com/articles/321484#ratios

https://www.urmc.rochester.edu/encyclopedia/content.aspx?ContentTypeID=16 7&ContentID=lipid_panel_hdl_ratio

https://www.nhs.uk/conditions/high-cholesterol/cholesterol-levels/

https://bmccardiovascdisord.biomedcentral.com/articles/10.1186/s12872-019-1228-7

CHAPTER 6: ADVANCED LIPIDS PROFILE

An advanced lipids profile is available privately or via a lipid clinic and should include some, or all, of:

- Small Dense LDL (sdLDL)
- Lipoprotein-A1 (Lp(a))
- Apolipoprotein A-1 (APO-A1)
- Apolipoprotein B (APO-B)
- Apolipoprotein C-II (APO-CII)
- Apolipoprotein C-III (APO-CIII)
- Apolipoprotein D (APO-D)
- Apolipoprotein E (APO-E)

Small dense LDL cholesterol - sdLDL

LDL particles vary in density, size, and chemical composition, and are divided into two main subtypes: small dense LDL (sdLDL) and large buoyant LDL (lbLDL). The sdLDL subtypes are smaller in size but higher in density, with a greater risk of penetrating the arterial wall. They are more susceptible to oxidation, remain in circulation longer (decreased affinity for LDL receptors), and have a longer half-life than other LDL particles, all of which contributes to their greater potential for causing atherosclerotic cardiovascular disease. As such, sdLDL levels are a better marker for cardiovascular disease prediction than total LDL.

If sdLDL has not been tested directly it can be estimated using the Sampson Equation which uses Total Cholesterol, HDL, and triglycerides to estimate levels of VLDL, LDL, lbLDL, as well as sdLDL.

The spreadsheet can be downloaded from:

https://figshare.com/articles/software/Sampson_sdLDLC_Equation_Calculator_xlsx/12888293

When using this spreadsheet, make sure you convert your values from mmol/L to mg/dL using a suitable conversion system, e.g. UnitsLab.com.

Raised sdLDL

Increased levels may be associated with:

- Dietary carbohydrate intake (fructose more so than glucose)
- Raised triglycerides
- Poorly managed diabetes
- Metabolic syndrome
- Infections
- Inflammation

Decreased sdLDL

Low levels may be associated with:

- Niacin
- Omega 3
- Exercise
- Medications: statins, fibrates, ezetimibe

sdLDL Reference Range

sdLDL is measured in milligrams per decilitre (mg/dL)

- Normal Range: <36mg/dL

References

https://www.optimaldx.com/research-blog/cardiovascular-biomarkers-small-dense-ldl-cholesterol

https://www.ncbi.nlm.nih.gov/books/NBK541036/

https://pubmed.ncbi.nlm.nih.gov/15539965/

https://pubmed.ncbi.nlm.nih.gov/11472706/

https://www.ncbi.nlm.nih.gov/pmc/articles/PMC3689018/

https://lipidworld.biomedcentral.com/articles/10.1186/s12944-022-01686-y

https://www.aacc.org/science-and-research/scientific-shorts/2021/small-dense-ldl-cholesterol-can-it-be-calculated

https://www.ncbi.nlm.nih.gov/pmc/articles/PMC8260186/

https://www.ncbi.nlm.nih.gov/pmc/articles/PMC5441126/

https://pubmed.ncbi.nlm.nih.gov/33876239/

https://www.ncbi.nlm.nih.gov/pmc/articles/PMC9025822/

https://www.ncbi.nlm.nih.gov/pmc/articles/PMC8866335

Lipoprotein (a) – Lp(a)

Levels of this lipoprotein are primarily determined by your genetics, and remain consistent through life, although secondary causes include chronic kidney disease, nephrotic kidney disease, and hypothyroidism.

This marker is not routinely tested but may be available via referral to a lipid clinic if there is a family history of cardiovascular disease or raised Lp(a), familial hypercholesterolaemia, calcific aortic valve disease, or a raised 10-year risk of cardiovascular disease.

If referral to a lipid clinic is not an option, testing may be available through private laboratories, e.g. with Randox Laboratories or The Doctors Laboratory.

Levels of Lp(a) may be raised even if LDL is low. Statins do not impact Lp(a) levels but new medications that work on Lp(a) levels from a genetic level are being researched. PCSK9 inhibitors may reduce Lp(a) but are not currently licensed for this use. In individuals with recurrent cardiovascular disease, lipoprotein apheresis (filtering LDL, Lp(a), and triglycerides from the blood) may reduce Lp(a) levels by up to 75%.

If an individual has raised Lp(a), refer them to their doctor to rule out secondary causes where appropriate, and then follow the suggestions in Chapter 10: Modifiable Diet and Lifestyle Risk Factors.

Raised Lp(a)

Increased levels of Lp(a) maybe associated with:

- o Atherosclerotic cardiovascular disease
- o Increase in blood clot development and strokes
- o Aortic stenosis (disease of the heart valve)
- o Alcohol consumption

Decreased Lp(a)

Decreased levels of Lp(a) do not appear to be clinically relevant, but may be associated with:

- o Aspirin usage
- o Niacin supplementation
- o Combined oestrogen and progestin therapy e.g. HRT

Lp(a) Reference Range

Lp(a) is measured in milligrams per litre (mg/L).

- Optimal Range: <140mg/L
- Borderline risk of cardiovascular disease: 140-300mg/L
- Increased risk of cardiovascular disease: 310-500mg/L
- Significantly elevated risk of cardiovascular disease: >500mg/L

References

https://cdnsciencepub.com/doi/10.1139/cjpp-2014-0478
https://www.heartuk.org.uk/genetic-conditions/high-lipoproteina
https://www.ncbi.nlm.nih.gov/books/NBK570621/

Apolipoprotein A-1 – APO-A1

APO-A1 is a protein encoded by the APOA1 gene that forms a major component of HDL particles in plasma. It is synthesised in hepatocytes and released to accumulate cholesterol from cells to form HDL particles. There are variable numbers of APO-A1 per HDL particle, so APO-A1 is not used as an alternative for measuring HDL levels.

In my bus analogy in chapter 1 APO-A1 was the bus driver of HDL, accepting passengers. In the bloodstream it is the protein on the surface of the HDL that activates enzymes to facilitate the uptake of cholesterol into the HDL.

Note: APO-A1 levels are not routinely used in analysis of atherosclerotic cardiovascular disease as evidence is conflicting.

Genetic mutations are associated with deficiencies of APO-A1 and HDL deficiencies and appears to correlate with an increased risk of atherosclerotic cardiovascular disease. However, APOA1-milano is an APOA1 genetic mutation found in Italy with individuals displaying low HDL but not increased risk of heart disease.

It is also possible to have adequate levels of HDL, but insufficient levels of APO-A1 to activate the enzymes to load the cholesterol into the HDL.

Raised APO-A1

Increased levels of APO-A1 may be associated with:

- Physical exercise
- Losing weight
- Pregnancy
- Niacin
- Medications – carbamazepine, oestrogens and OCP, phenytoin, fibrates, ethanol, phenobarbital, some statins (lovastatin, pravastatin, simvastatin)
- Genetics – familial hyperalphalipoproteinaemia, familial cholesteryl ester transfer protein deficiency

Decreased APO-A1

Low levels of APO-A1 may be associated with:

- Chronic kidney failure
- Nephrotic syndrome
- Smoking
- Poorly controlled diabetes
- Coronary artery disease (narrowed and hardened arteries)
- Liver disease
- Cholestasis
- Medications: androgens, progestins, beta blockers, diuretics
- Genetics: hypoalphalipoproteinaemia, Tangier disease

APO-A1 Reference Range

APO-A1 is measured in milligrams per decilitre (mg/dL)

- Normal Male Range: 110-180mg/dL
- Normal Female Range: 110-205mg/dL

Low APO-A1, particularly in the presence of raised APO-B would suggest an increased risk of atherosclerotic cardiovascular disease.

References:

https://labtestsonline.org.uk/tests/apo

https://healthmatters.io/understand-blood-test-results/apolipoprotein-1

https://www.thelancet.com/journals/lancet/article/PIIS0140-6736(08)61076-4/fulltext

https://www.urmc.rochester.edu/encyclopedia/content.aspx?contenttypeid=167&contentid=apolipoprotein_a

Apolipoprotein B – APO-B

APO-B is a protein encoded by the APOB gene that forms a major component of chylomicrons, VLDL, LDL, IDL, and Lp(a) particles in plasma, and plays a key role in lipid transport and metabolism.

APO-B48 is synthesised in the intestines and forms an integral part of the structure of chylomicrons, transporting dietary lipids from the intestines to the liver. Here, the liver repackages the chylomicrons and combines them with APO-B100 to form VLDL, which later becomes IDL and then LDL via the action of the lipoprotein lipase enzyme.

Lab tests generally only report APO-B, and unless otherwise specified, this is APO-B100 as there is no known clinical need to measure APO-B48 at this time. Research is suggesting that APO-B is a more reliable marker for assessing risk of atherosclerotic cardiovascular disease than LDL, or non-HDL, as there is one APO-B per lipoprotein.

Raised APO-B

Increased levels of APO-B may be associated with:

- Uncontrolled diabetes
- Alcohol intake
- Hypothyroidism
- Nephrotic syndrome

- Pregnancy
- Hepatic obstruction
- Cushing's syndrome
- Medications: androgens, beta blockers, diuretics, progestins, corticosteroids, catecholamines
- Genetics: familial hypercholesterolaemia

Decreased APO-B

Low levels of APO-B may be associated with:

- Hyperthyroidism
- Malnutrition or malabsorption of nutrients
- Reye's syndrome
- Weight loss
- Following severe illness or surgery
- Cirrhosis of the liver
- Niacin
- Medications: oestrogens, statins, thyroxine
- Genetics: familial hypobetalipoproteinaemia

APO-B Reference Range

APO-B is measured in milligrams per decilitre (mg/dL).

- Normal Range: <100mg/dL

References

https://www.pritikin.com/what-is-apob
https://labtestsonline.org.uk/tests/apo-b
https://www.ncbi.nlm.nih.gov/books/NBK538139

APO-B:APO-A1 ratio

The APO-B:APO-A1 ratio is used to evaluate the risk of atherosclerotic cardiovascular disease and has a strong correlation with myocardial infarction rates.

The ratio reflects the balance between APO-B rich particles (chylomicrons, VLDL, IDL, LDL, Lp(a)) and APO-A1 particles (HDL).

The formula to calculate the APO-B:APO-A1 ratio is:

$$APO\text{-}B \div APO\text{-}A1 = APO\text{-}B\text{:}APO\text{-}A1$$

Raised APO-B:APO-A1 Ratio

An increased ratio is associated with an increased risk of atherosclerotic cardiovascular disease, myocardial infarction, and metabolic syndrome. In individuals with existing atherosclerotic cardiovascular disease, an increased ratio is associated with increased severity of the cardiovascular disease and poorer outcomes. In this way, the ratio can be used to identify those who require additional lifestyle modifications or disease monitoring.

Decreased APO-B:APO-A1 Ratio

A decreased ratio is associated with lower risk of atherosclerotic cardiovascular disease.

APO-B:APO-A1 Reference Range

As APO-B:APO-A1 is a ratio, there are no units.

- Normal Range: <0.9
- Increased risk of metabolic syndrome: >0.85 in men (0.8 women)
- Increased risk of cardiovascular disease: >0.9

References

https://www.thelancet.com/journals/lancet/article/PIIS0140-6736(08)61076-4/fulltext

https://www.ncbi.nlm.nih.gov/pmc/articles/PMC4380097/

https://www.thelancet.com/journals/lancet/article/PIIS0140-6736(08)61076-4/fulltext

https://lipidworld.biomedcentral.com/articles/10.1186/1476-511X-13-81

https://lipidworld.biomedcentral.com/articles/10.1186/s12944-019-1144-y

https://www.thelancet.com/journals/ebiom/article/PIIS2352-3964(21)00036-0/fulltext

Apolipoprotein CII – APO-CII

APO-CII is a protein encoded by the APOC2 gene that forms a major part of VLDL and chylomicrons. It is a co-factor for activating the lipoprotein lipase (LPL) enzyme, which facilitates the regulation of triglycerides in the blood by liberating them from chylomicrons and VLDL.

Mutations of the APOC2 gene should be investigated in individuals who present with hypertriglyceridaemia, xanthomas, pancreatitis, abdominal pain, and hepatosplenomegaly. These individuals may also have an increased risk of early atherosclerosis, reflected in their raised triglycerides and cholesterol levels.

Decreased APO-CII

Low levels of APO-CII may be associated with:

- Hyperlipoproteinaemia type IB
- Familial LPL deficiency (high TGs)
- Familial apolipoprotein CII deficiency

Absence of APO-CII

Mutations leading to a total absence of APO-CII on protein electrophoresis is mainly treated with a fat-free diet.

APO-CII Reference Range

APO-CII is reported in milligrams per decilitre (mg/dL) but may also be reported simply as Present / Absent

- Normal Range: 1.6-4.2mg/dL

References

Reference range: Randox laboratory

https://www.cancertherapyadvisor.com/home/decision-support-in-medicine/labmed/familial-apolipoprotein-cii-deficiency/

https://pubmed.ncbi.nlm.nih.gov/31477272

https://www.ncbi.nlm.nih.gov/gene?Db=gene&Cmd=ShowDetailView&TermToSearch=344

https://patient.info/doctor/apolipoproteins

Apolipoprotein CIII – APO-CIII

APO-CIII is a protein encoded by the APOC3 gene that forms a major part of triglyceride-rich lipoproteins – chylomicrons, VLDL, and IDL. It also forms part of some HDL and may negatively influence those HDL's association with cardiovascular disease.

APO-CIII inhibits the lipoprotein lipase enzyme and hepatic lipase, which inhibits the liberation of triglycerides from the lipoproteins.

Raised APO-CIII

Increased levels of APO-CIII may result in hypertriglyceridaemia, an increased risk of coronary artery calcification, and there may be an association with non-alcoholic fatty liver disease (NAFLD)

Decreased APO-CIII

Low levels of APO-CIII may be seen in individuals with stomach cancer.

APO-CIII Reference Range

APO-CIII is measured in milligrams per decilitre (mg/dL).

- Normal Range: 5.5-9.5mg/dL

References

Randox labs for reference range

https://www.ncbi.nlm.nih.gov/pmc/articles/PMC4556282/
https://www.ncbi.nlm.nih.gov/pmc/articles/PMC3090227/
https://www.ncbi.nlm.nih.gov/pmc/articles/PMC5916256/
https://www.sciencedirect.com/topics/neuroscience/apolipoprotein-c3

Apolipoprotein D – APO-D

APO-D is a protein encoded by the APOD gene that forms a component of HDL, with evidence suggesting that it may support the antioxidant and anti-inflammatory activities of HDL.

Raised levels of APO-D may be associated with androgen insensitivity syndrome.

Apolipoprotein E – APO-E

APO-E is a protein encoded by the APOE gene, and the protein encoded by this gene forms a part of VLDL and IDL, facilitating their clearance from the plasma via APO-E receptor recognition in the liver.

APO-E is also found as part of a subtype of HDL.

There are three common isoforms, or alleles of the APOE gene (APOE2, APOE3, APOE4) each carrying different risks for Alzheimer's disease and cardiovascular disease:

Absent or Mutated APO-E

Absent or mutated APO-E may be associated with:

- Familial dysbetalipoproteinaemia
- Hyperlipoproteinaemia type III
- Alzheimer's (APO-E4)
- Hypercholesterolaemia (APO-E4)
- Peripheral vascular disease (APO-E2)

- Thromboembolism (APO-E2)
- Arterial aneurysm (APO-E2)
- Peptic ulcer (APO-E2)
- Cervical disorders (APO-E2)

References:

https://patient.info/doctor/apolipoproteins

https://www.nature.com/articles/269604a0

https://www.ahajournals.org/doi/abs/10.1161/01.atv.8.1.1

https://www.ncbi.nlm.nih.gov/pmc/articles/PMC2674716/

https://pubmed.ncbi.nlm.nih.gov/3283935/

https://www.frontiersin.org/articles/10.3389/fcell.2021.635527/full

CHAPTER 7: ADDITIONAL RISK MARKERS FOR CARDIOVASCULAR DISEASE

When working with a client with raised lipids, or other risk factors associated with cardiovascular disease e.g. raised blood pressure or diabetes, the following markers should also be considered. Some will be easily available through the client's doctor, while others may require private testing.

- High Sensitivity C-Reactive Protein (HS-CRP)
- Erythrocyte Sedimentation Rate (ESR)
- Glycated Haemoglobin (HbA1C)
- Fasting Insulin
- C-Peptide
- Fasting Glucose
- HOMA-IR score
- Alanine Transaminase (ALT) & Aspartate Transaminase (AST)
- Serum Ferritin
- Uric Acid
- Lactate Dehydrogenase
- Homocysteine
- B6, B9, B12
- Vitamin D

High Sensitivity C-Reactive Protein – HS-CRP

HS-CRP produced in the liver as a product of interleukin-6, interleukin-1B, and tumor necrosis factor alpha. These inflammatory markers, together with other inflammatory markers, and substances from arteries, adipose tissue, inflamed tissues, infections, autoimmune diseases (lupus, RA), bacteria, cancer, burns, and more are processed into HS-CRP in the liver. As such, HS-CRP is a marker of inflammation (though not the cause of inflammation itself) and raised levels are associated with predicting cardiovascular disease in healthy individuals with no previous history of cardiovascular disease or predicting recurrent cardiovascular events and mortality in individuals with pre-existing cardiovascular disease.

Any infection may cause a temporary increase in HS-CRP – even a sore throat, H.Pylori, periodontal disease, sinusitis etc. so infection should be ruled out when initially looking at a raised HS-CRP result. Often a doctor will retest a raised HS-CRP after a set period to rule out infection as a temporary cause of raised levels.

HS-CRP promotes inflammation, oxidative stress, and autoimmune disfunction in many ways, including through activation of complement pathways, influence on lipids uptake by macrophages, and inhibition of nitric oxide production promoting endothelial dysfunction.

The raised sensitivity of HS-CRP is better than the traditional CRP for detecting the low level of long-term inflammation in the arteries from atherosclerosis, but unfortunately, HS-CRP is not widely available with all doctors. Although the HS-CRP test measures even trace amounts of CRP in the blood and is therefore more sensitive than a CRP test, the CRP test is still a reasonable test for detecting inflammation in the body.

HS-CRP is non-specific and may be elevated in any inflammatory condition, so a raised HS-CRP does not necessarily equal a higher risk of heart attack.

Raised HS-CRP

Increased levels of HS-CRP may be associated with:

- Infection
- Inflammation

Decreased HS-CRP

Low levels of HS-CRP are not clinically relevant.

HS-CRP Reference Range

- Low cardiovascular risk: <1mg/L
- Moderate cardiovascular risk: 1-3mg/L
- High cardiovascular risk: >3mg/L

Note: if LDL is >4.1mmol/L and HS-CRP is raised >1mg/L, further investigations and lifestyle interventions should be made.

References

https://www.sciencedirect.com/science/article/pii/S1110260814001173

https://pubmed.ncbi.nlm.nih.gov/15258556/

https://www.sciencedirect.com/science/article/abs/pii/S014628060400074X?via%3Dihub

Erythrocyte Sedimentation Rate – ESR

ESR is a marker of how quickly red blood cells (erythrocytes) in the blood sample settle at the bottom of a test tube in one hour. Normally the blood cells will settle slowly, but if they settle faster there may be inflammation, and the reading will be raised within the one-hour time frame.

A raised ESR may indicate inflammation in the body, caused by an infection, an injury, chronic disease, or an autoimmune disorder; or it may indicate other medical conditions such as arthritis, IBD, and cancers.

Inflammation causes changes to the physiology of the RBC membranes, resulting in them clumping together and settling at a faster rate of millimetres per hour.

As a side note, ESR can be measured manually over the 1-hour time frame in Westergren tubes, or the measurement can be automated.

Raised ESR

In the presence of cardiovascular disease, raised ESR would support the inflammatory aetiology of cardiovascular disease in a client, and was found to be a strong predictor of cardiovascular disease mortality.

Decreased ESR

A lower ESR is generally clinically insignificant, unless associated with an increased white blood cell count, increased red blood cell count, or sickle cell anaemia.

ESR Reference Range

ESR is measured in millimetres per hour (mm/h).

- Optimal Male Range: <5mm/h
- Optimal Female Range: <10mm/h

References

https://www.ncbi.nlm.nih.gov/pmc/articles/PMC3333472/

Glycated Haemoglobin – HbA1C

HbA1C is a form of haemoglobin within a red blood cell that has chemically joined to a monosaccharide (glucose, galactose, and fructose) in the blood, in a process known as glycation.

The amount of monosaccharide that binds to the haemoglobin is directly proportional to the total amount of sugar in the body at that time, and the average lifespan of a red blood cell is 8-12 weeks, so HbA1C is used to provide a two to three-month average blood sugar level and can be used to assess for possible insulin resistance.

Raised HbA1C

Raised blood sugar levels over several weeks will be echoed in a raised HbA1C test.

Raised HbA1C levels indicate an increased risk of all-cause mortality, cardiovascular disease, and cardiovascular disease mortality, particularly in individuals under 55 years of age. It may also be raised due to diabetes mellitus, kidney failure, blood loss, increased red blood cell turnover and other red blood cell disorders.

Decreased HbA1C

Decreased HbA1C may indicate a well-controlled client dietary intake, excessive use of antidiabetic drugs, haemolytic anaemia, or haemorrhage.

HbA1C Reference Range

HbA1C may be measured in millimoles per mole (mmol/mol) or as a percentage.

- Optimal Range: <37mmol/mol (<5.5%)
- Normal Range: <42mmol/mol (<6.0%)
- Pre-diabetic Range: 42 to 47 mmol/mol (6.0%-6.4%)
- Diabetes: >48mmol/mol (>6.5%)

References

https://cardiab.biomedcentral.com/articles/10.1186/s12933-021-01413-4
https://www.ncbi.nlm.nih.gov/pmc/articles/PMC5642750/

Fasting Insulin

Insulin is a hormone produced initially in the beta cells of the pancreas as preproinsulin that is cleaved twice to become insulin, and then proinsulin and C-Peptide. Insulin facilitates the transport of glucose into the cells of the body, thereby maintaining normal blood glucose levels. Without insulin, blood glucose levels would raise, eventually leading to diabetic coma.

Too much insulin for the blood glucose is known as hyperinsulinaemia, which can lead to hypoglycaemia (low blood glucose levels).

Too little insulin for the blood glucose is known as hypoinsulinaemia, which can lead to hyperglycaemia (high blood glucose levels).

When the body becomes resistant to insulin, high blood sugars develop (often referred to as pre-diabetes) which contributes to cardiovascular disease as the hyperglycaemic levels trigger oxidative stress and inflammatory response, leading to cellular damage. Additional contributions to cardiovascular disease from insulin resistance include its influence on lipid metabolism leading to raised plasma triglycerides, low HDL, and an increase of sdLDL, and its role in endothelial dysfunction.

Raised fasting insulin

Increased levels of insulin when fasting may be associated with:

- Acromegaly
- Cushing's
- Fructose or galactose intolerance
- Insulinomas
- Obesity
- Insulin resistance (if insulin raised and glucose normal/moderately raised)
- Type 2 diabetes
- Medications: corticosteroids, levodopa, OCP

Decreased fasting insulin

Low levels of fasting insulin may be associated with:

- Type 1 diabetes
- Hypopituitarism
- Inadequate calorie intake
- Over-exercising without recovery
- Low carb, high fat diet

Insulin Reference Range

Insulin is measured in micro international units per millilitre (µIU/mL or uIU/mL) and should always be tested when fasting.

- Normal Range: <10µIU/mL
- Optimal Range: 2-6µIU/mL
- Hyperinsulinaemia / Possible Insulin Resistance: >8µIU/mL

Note: A particularly poor picture would be raised/normal insulin levels together with raised c-peptide, raised sdLDL, and a positive insulin tolerance test (ITT – an IV of insulin followed by insulin and glucose tests).

If insulin levels are below 2, together with raised blood glucose levels or HbA1C >44mmol/L, type 1 diabetes and LADA should be ruled out by a doctor.

References

https://www.levelshealth.com/blog/what-are-normal-insulin-levels-and-why-dont-we-test-it-more

https://thebloodcode.com/homa-ir-know/

https://academic.oup.com/eurheartj/article/41/Supplement_2/ehaa946.3057/606022

https://cardiab.biomedcentral.com/articles/10.1186/s12933-018-0762-4

https://labtestsonline.org.uk/tests/insulin

C-Peptide

While making insulin, the pancreas also produces C-Peptide. Both insulin and C-Peptide are released into the bloodstream, but C-Peptide does not influence blood sugar levels and is easier to measure as it stays in the bloodstream for longer. In this way, C-Peptide can be used to assess how much insulin is being produced and whether that insulin is being used effectively.

Over time C-Peptide degrades and is removed from the bloodstream by the kidneys.

In clients without diabetes, raised C-Peptide may be associated with decreased HDL, and increased risk of cardiovascular disease.

Testing for C-Peptide must be done with a fasted sample.

Raised C-Peptide

Increased C-Peptide levels may be associated with:

- Insulin resistance
- Type 2 diabetes
- Raised insulin levels (overproduction, or insulin resistance)
- Insulinomas
- Hypokalaemia
- Pregnancy
- Cushing's syndrome
- Kidney disease

- Lack of exercise
- Medications: glucocorticoids, sulfonylureas (for increasing insulin production)

Raised C-Peptide results may also be seen with an increased score on a coronary arterial calcium scan (CACS) and is associated with increased cardiovascular disease mortality rate.

Decreased C-Peptide

Low levels of C-Peptide may be associated with:

- Type 1 diabetes
- Latent autoimmune diabetes in adults (LADA)
- High dose biotin
- Alcohol consumption
- Excessive fasting
- Pancreatitis or pancreatectomy
- Hypoglycaemia from insulin injections
- Medications: diuretics

C-Peptide Reference Range

C-Peptide is measured in micrograms per millilitre (mcg/mL) and should always be measured when fasted.

- Normal Range (fasted): 0.8-3.85mcg/mL
- Normal Range (post-prandial): 3-9mcg/mL

Note: Levels of C-Peptide below 0.6mcg/mL may indicate possible beta cell failure e.g. Type 1 diabetes.

References:

https://pubmed.ncbi.nlm.nih.gov/25782584/

https://www.ncbi.nlm.nih.gov/pmc/articles/PMC3680586/

https://labs.selfdecode.com/blog/c-peptide

https://pubmed.ncbi.nlm.nih.gov/29392827/

https://ncbi.nlm.nih.gov/pmc/articles/PMC3000615/

https://pubmed.ncbi.nlm.nih.gov/3909371/

https://www.ncbi.nlm.nih.gov/pmc/articles/PMC4283961

https://labtestsonline.org.uk/tests/c-peptide

Fasting Glucose

Carbohydrates in the diet are digested to produce glucose. Insulin is then secreted by the pancreas to transport the glucose out of the bloodstream and into the cells to maintain homeostasis of the blood glucose levels. Excess glucose spikes require repeated insulin secretions. Eventually, the cells become less sensitive to insulin and require more insulin to maintain the normal blood glucose levels, leading to consistently raised blood glucose levels, insulin resistance, pre-diabetes, and finally diabetes.

Glucose is often tested in preference to insulin as testing methods for insulin are not standardised, and consistent reference ranges have not been set. Sadly, raised glucose levels may only be seen after several years of raised insulin levels meaning that not testing insulin levels delays prediction of future health issues.

Raised Fasting Glucose

Increased fasting glucose levels may be associated with:

- Insulin resistance
- Type 1 diabetes
- Type 2 diabetes
- Latent autoimmune diabetes in adults (LADA)
- Gestational diabetes
- Overweight
- High blood pressure

- Heart attack
- Stroke
- Genetics

Decreased Fasting Glucose

Low levels of fasting glucose levels may be associated with:

- Hypoglycaemia
- Medications: diabetes medications e.g. metformin, GLP-1 and dual GLP-1/GIP receptor agonists, SGLT2 inhibitors, sulfonylureas, thiazolidinediones, alpha-glucosidase inhibitors, bile acid sequestrants

Glucose Reference Range

Glucose is measured in milligrams per decilitre (mg/dL) and should always be tested when fasting:

- Hypoglycaemic Range: <70mg/dL (3.9mmol/L)
- Normal Range: 70mg/dL (3.9mmol/L)- 100mg/dL (5.6mmol/L)
- Pre-diabetic Range: 100mg/dL – 125mg/dL (5.6-6.9mmol/L) consider changes to diet and lifestyle
- Diabetes: 126mg/dL (7mmol/L) on more than 2 separate blood tests

References

https://www.who.int/data/gho/indicator-metadata-registry/imr-details/2380

https://www.levelshealth.com/blog/what-are-normal-insulin-levels-and-why-dont-we-test-it-more

https://diabetes.org/healthy-living/medication-treatments/oral-other-injectable-diabetes-medications

HOMA-IR score

HOMA-IR stands for Homeostatic Model Assessment of Insulin Resistance and is a calculation that may be used to assess the presence and extent of any insulin resistance.

The formula to calculate HOMA-IR will vary based on whether your fasting glucose is in nmol/L or mg/dL.

If you have fasting glucose in nmol/L, then the formula for calculating HOMA-IR is:

Fasting Insulin x (Fasting Glucose / 22.5)

Example calculation:

Fasting insulin 3.5uU/L

Fasting glucose 4.5mmol/L

= 3.5 x (4.5 / 22.5) = 0.7 = HOMA-IR

If you have fasting glucose in mg/dL, then the calculation for HOMA-IR is:

(Fasting Insulin x Fasting Glucose) / 405

Example calculation:

Fasting insulin: 3.5uU/L

Fasting glucose: 85mg/dL

= (3.5 x 85) / 405 = 0.73 = HOMA-IR

Raised HOMA-IR

A raised HOMA-IR score indicates insulin resistance – the higher the reading, the more resistant the cells are to insulin, indicating that dietary and lifestyle changes are required.

Decreased HOMA-IR

A low HOMA-IR score indicates that cells are sensitive to insulin, and this is the optimal state.

HOMA-IR Reference Range

There are no units for the result of the HOMA-IR calculation.

- Insulin sensitive: <1 (optimal)
- Early insulin resistance: >1.9
- Significant insulin resistance: >2.9

References

https://pubmed.ncbi.nlm.nih.gov/20721461

https://healthunlocked.com/diabetesindia/posts/145008445/homo-ir-test-for-insulin-resistance

https://thebloodcode.com/homa-ir-know/

Alanine Transaminase & Aspartate Transaminase – ALT & AST

These enzymes are produced in the liver and found in high levels in the bloodstream when there is damage to the liver. Studies have observed raised ALT and AST levels correlating with insulin resistance (raised HOMA-IR scores) in patients with early (undetected) NAFLD. NAFLD is normally not diagnosed until liver enzymes are 1-2 times the upper reference range (e.g. around 100-150U/L)

Note that ALT can vary up to 45% in any one day, with values being raised in afternoons, so I would strongly recommend looking at more than one set of blood results before drawing any conclusions.

ALT & AST Reference Range

Both ALT and AST are measured in units per litre (U/L).

- Optimal Range: 10-20U/L

References

https://www.ncbi.nlm.nih.gov/pmc/articles/PMC6499277

https://www.thieme-connect.com/products/ejournals/abstract/10.1055/a-0603-7899

https://pubmed.ncbi.nlm.nih.gov/29723898/

https://www.ncbi.nlm.nih.gov/books/NBK482489/

Serum Ferritin

Ferritin is a protein that stores iron, and only releases it when your body needs it. Very little ferritin circulates in your blood, but instead it is mostly found in the liver, bone marrow, muscles, and spleen. When the body needs more red blood cells, a signal from the body triggers cells in these locations to release ferritin, which in turn binds with transferrin to transport it to where new red blood cells are made.

Ferritin is also a positive acute phase protein and levels will rise significantly when there is inflammation, making it a useful marker of acute and chronic inflammation. It is a non-specific marker, meaning that it may raise for a range of inflammatory conditions including rheumatoid arthritis, acute infections, malignancy, diabetes, and cardiovascular disease.

Serum Ferritin Reference Range

Serum ferritin is measured in micrograms per litre (mcg/L).

- Optimal Range: 70-100mcg/L (m); 70-90mcg/L (f)
- Alarm range: >300mcg/L

Ferritin may also be raised with primary/secondary iron overload (e.g. haemochromatosis, or excess iron infusions/supplements). If ferritin is raised, it would be wise to test a full iron panel to rule out primary/secondary iron overload. This is covered in my book, Blood Labs 1.

References

https://www.ncbi.nlm.nih.gov/pmc/articles/PMC2893236

https://www.ncbi.nlm.nih.gov/pmc/articles/PMC3767354/

Uric acid

Uric acid is commonly associated with gout, a type of arthritis whereby urate crystals accumulate in the joints due to raised levels of uric acid. However, raised uric acid (hyperuricaemia) is also considered a risk factor in the development of cardiovascular disease including hypertension, coronary artery disease, and cardiovascular mortality, as well as promoting impaired glucose tolerance and insulin resistance.

Raised uric acid is associated with diets high in sugar and alcohol, so the suggestions made in Chapter 10: Modifiable Diet and Lifestyle Risk Factors should be reviewed.

Uric Acid Reference Range

Uric acid is measured in micromoles per litre (umol/L).

- Normal Range: <357umol/L

References

https://www.sciencedirect.com/science/article/pii/S0914508720304159#

https://journals.plos.org/plosone/article?id=10.1371/journal.pone.0147737

Lactate Dehydrogenase – LDH

LDH is an enzyme found in many tissues and organs including muscles, liver, heart, pancreas, kidneys, brain, and blood cells. When raised levels are found in the blood stream there is an indication that there is tissue/organ damage somewhere, such as a muscle injury, heart attack, pancreatitis, or a disease affecting tissues such as autoimmunity, anaemia, kidney disease, liver disease, or an infection such as meningitis, encephalitis, or Epstein-Barr virus (glandular fever), or cancers such as lymphoma or leukaemia. Note that LDH is a generic marker and doesn't identify which organ may be damaged, or which disease or infection may be present.

Raised LDH levels may also be associated with arterial stiffness and subsequent increase of cardiovascular risk.

Strenuous exercise can also raise LDH temporarily as it is released from the muscles post-exercise. Raised platelet levels will result in an artificially raised LDH level being reported that does not reflect the actual level of LDH present.

Haemolysed blood samples will result in falsely raised LDH being reported.

LDH Reference Range

Lactate dehydrogenase is measured in international units per litre (IU/L).

- Normal Range: 140-280U/L

References

https://www.ncbi.nlm.nih.gov/pmc/articles/PMC8742599/

https://onlinelibrary.wiley.com/doi/pdf/10.1016/S1388-9842(02)00088-0

https://www.urmc.rochester.edu/encyclopedia/content.aspx?contenttypeid=167&contentid=lactic_acid_dehydrogenase_blood

https://www.ncbi.nlm.nih.gov/books/NBK557536/

Homocysteine

Homocysteine is currently difficult to test privately outside London (do let me know if you find a lab offering it to practitioners at an affordable price, and/or the public, outside London!) and is not routinely tested with the NHS at this time though may be available via a lipid clinic or haematologist.

Homocysteine is a common amino acid found in the blood as a by-product of the conversion of methionine from meat consumption. Homocysteine may be recycled into methionine with B12 and folate as co-factors, and into cysteine/glutathione with B6 as a co-factor.

Raised homocysteine (hyperhomocysteinaemia) is a mediator in the formation of cardiovascular disease through various mechanisms, including damaging arterial endothelium and smooth muscle cells, promoting endothelial dysfunction and oxidative damage.

Raised Homocysteine

Increased levels of homocysteine are associated with:

- Poor diet and/or excess consumption of meat
- Kidney disease
- Thyroid dysfunction
- Cancer
- Psoriasis
- Diabetes

- Menopause
- Older age
- Drugs, tobacco, and alcohol
- Being male
- Nutrient deficiencies: B6, B9, B12
- Medications: any that affect B6, B9, or B12 metabolism

Raised serum creatinine can also raise homocysteine levels.

Support diet and lifestyle (see Chapter 10: Modifiable Diet and Lifestyle Risk Factors) to lower homocysteine and consequent cardiovascular risk.

Decreased Homocysteine

Low levels of homocysteine may be caused by MTHFR genetic mutations affecting methylation pathways.

Homocysteine Reference Range

Homocysteine is measured in micromoles per litre (umol/L).

- Insufficient homocysteine for glutathione production: <7umol/L
- Optimal Range: 7-9umol/L
- Raised: >15umol/L

References

https://www.seekinghealth.com/blogs/education/what-is-homocysteine

https://www.ncbi.nlm.nih.gov/pmc/articles/PMC4326479

https://www.webmd.com/heart-disease/guide/homocysteine-risk

Folic Acid (B9), B6, B12 – for homocysteine

Low levels of these b vitamins may be associated with raised homocysteine, as they are required for the conversion of homocysteine to methionine (B9, B12) and cysteine (B6).

B9 and B12 are covered in detail in my book, Blood Labs 1.

Simply supplementing B6, B9, and B12 to lower homocysteine levels does not appear to reduce risk of cardiovascular disease – the environment still needs to be supported, and this is covered in Chapter 10: Modifiable Diet and Lifestyle Risk Factors.

B9 Reference Range

Serum folate may be expressed as nanograms per millilitre (ng/mL) or nanomoles per litre (nmol/L).

- Optimal Range: 12-17ng/mL (27-38.5nmol/L)

B12 Reference Range

B12 may be expressed as picomoles per litre, or nanograms per millilitre (ng/L).

- Optimal Range: 700-1000pmol/L (948-1355ng/L)

Vitamin D

Known as "the sunshine vitamin", vitamin D is a fat-soluble vitamin made from ultraviolet rays from sunlight striking exposing unprotected skin and triggering vitamin D synthesis (a process that also requires cholesterol).

It may also be found in small amounts in foods such as egg yolk, fortified cereals/foods, and fatty fish.

Vitamin D obtained from sunlight, food sources, or supplements needs to be converted to active vitamin D via two hydroxylation processes in the body - the first happens in the liver, and the second in the kidneys.

In some studies, individuals with lower vitamin D levels have an increased likelihood of raised cholesterol levels, although supplementing with vitamin D provides mixed results in terms of raising/decreasing cholesterol levels.

Vitamin D is covered in detail in my book, Blood Labs 1.

Vitamin D Reference Range

Serum concentrations of 25(OH)D may be reported in both nanomoles per litre (nmol/L) and nanograms per millilitre (ng/mL).

- Males & Females: >75nmol/L (>30ng/mL)

CHAPTER 8: CARDIOVASCULAR RISK CALCULATORS

QRISK® 3

QRISK®3 is an algorithm model used to estimate a 10-year risk of cardiovascular disease. It was first published in 2007 (QRISK®) and was updated in 2008 (QRISK®2) and 2017 (QRISK®3).

The results of the QRISK®3 calculator is only valid if there is no current diagnosis of cardiovascular disease, stroke, or transient ischaemic attack.

The result of the QRISK®3 algorithm may be estimated or actual.

Estimated QRISK®3 score: This means that some data was left blank, e.g. blood pressure. If your client has a raised estimated score, work with them to establish additional data to work towards an actual score. Free blood pressure measurements are available in some pharmacies, and they can request a lipid profile from their doctor if they have not had it tested before and are over 40 years old, if they are overweight or if cardiovascular disease/high cholesterol runs in the family.

Actual QRISK®3 Score: This means that all data was entered into the algorithm, leading to a more reliable prediction of cardiovascular disease.

In essence though, all scores are estimated as it's impossible to 100% predict the future of an individual's cardiovascular disease risk.

QRISK®3 does not take triglyceride levels into consideration.

The online QRISK®3 calculator can be found here: https://qrisk.org/

QRISK®3 Reference Range

- Low risk: QRISK®3 <10% (less than 1 in 10 chance of developing cardiovascular disease in the next 10 years)
- Moderate risk: QRISK®3 10-20% (1-2 in ten chance of developing cardiovascular disease in next 10 years)
- High risk: >20% (2 in 10 chance of developing cardiovascular disease in next 10 years)

NICE recommend that individuals with a score >10% should make changes to their lifestyle, diet, and consider Statin medications to lower cholesterol levels.

References

https://www.nhs.uk/conditions/high-cholesterol/getting-tested

https://www.bmj.com/content/357/bmj.j2099

https://www.nice.org.uk/guidance/cg181/resources/patient-decision-aid-pdf-243780159

https://www.hornchurchhealthcare.co.uk/appointmentstest-referrals/tests-investigations/cardiovascular-risk-score-qrisk3-patient-information-leaflet/

Framingham Risk Score

The Framingham Heart Study began between 1948 and 1952 with over 5000 participants whose health was reviewed every 2 years, and further participants have been enrolled since then. The study has been used to assess the connections between, among other things, smoking, high cholesterol, and high blood pressure.

A Framingham Risk Score is the result produced by an algorithm used to calculate the 10-year cardiovascular risk of an individual, based on the data collected in the Framingham Heart Study.

QRISK®3 is thought to be more accurate than the Framingham Risk Score, particularly for men, but the results of the Framingham Risk Score are still considered to be reliable.

You can access and use the calculator here: https://qxmd.com/calculate/calculator_252/framingham-risk-score-2008

JBS3 Heart Risk Calculator

No longer widely available for use, the JBS3 risk calculator aimed to calculate an individual's lifetime risk of cardiovascular disease and show the benefits of interventions on their particular risk of cardiovascular disease.

ASSIGN

Developed and used in Scotland, ASSIGN was designed in 2006 to calculate 10-year cardiovascular disease risk using not only the classic risk factors (total cholesterol, HDL cholesterol, Systolic BP, smoking status) for cardiovascular disease, but also including social deprivation (Scottish postcodes only) and family history of cardiovascular disease.

Try it here: https://www.assign-score.com/estimate-the-risk/

References

https://heart.bmj.com/content/100/Suppl_2/ii1

https://www.ncbi.nlm.nih.gov/pmc/articles/PMC5051389/

https://www.assign-score.com/

https://www.ncbi.nlm.nih.gov/pmc/articles/PMC4159698/

CHAPTER 9: COMMON CONDITIONS TO CONSIDER

Familial Hypercholesterolaemia (FH)

FH is a genetic mutation affecting the clearance of LDL cholesterol in the liver. It often goes undetected until routine lipid testing. Individuals with FH may present with tendon xanthomata, xanthelasma, or corneal arcus as visible symptoms, and are likely to have a family history of early cardiovascular disease.

Around 60-80% of people with FH have a mutation in one of these genes: LDLR, APOB, and PCSK9, and will present with LDL levels >5mmol/L.

Routine treatment is with statins or PCSK9 inhibitors, but a CAC scan will show whether statins are needed. Healthy lifestyle is key, and a diet low in saturated fats that reduces risk of obesity but may not be enough if levels are very high.

References

https://www.cdc.gov/genomics/disease/fh/FH.htm

Menopause

Menopause is considered to start 12 months after a woman's last menstrual cycle, and perimenopause is the period of time leading up to menopause. Blood tests and support for menopause is covered in my book, Bloods Labs 2.

Prior to menopause, women have a lower average rate of cardiovascular disease than men.

However, as oestrogen assists with the regulation of lipid metabolism in the liver, the drop in oestrogen levels associated with menopause leads to raised LDL and triglycerides, and the balance of HDL to non-HDL becomes less optimal. Entering menopause younger may increase risk of heart disease compared to women who enter menopause later in life.

Menopause is also associated with an increase of total and central adipose tissue and a decrease in insulin sensitivity, which will influence the metabolism of blood lipids.

Women who start HRT within 5 years of their last period are 20% more likely to have a coronary arterial calcium scan (CACS) of zero and, overall, HRT users are 30% less likely to die of other causes.

While HRT may be an option, it is still important to consider the full context as diet and lifestyle will still play a key role. HRT does not completely protect against cardiovascular disease but may protect against non-alcoholic fatty liver disease (NAFLD), insulin resistance, and type 2 diabetes. Oral oestrogen may raise triglycerides, which may offset the cardioprotective benefits of oestrogen.

References

https://thebms.org.uk/2017/03/hormone-replacement-therapy-can-lower-risk-early-death-women-new-study-suggests/

https://www.ncbi.nlm.nih.gov/pmc/articles/PMC5763482/

https://www.medicalnewstoday.com/articles/menopause-and-cholesterol

https://pubmed.ncbi.nlm.nih.gov/32187130/

https://www.jacc.org/doi/10.1016/S0735-1097%2817%2934797-6

https://www.ncbi.nlm.nih.gov/pmc/articles/PMC5258833/

https://www.cedars-sinai.org/newsroom/study-hormone-replacement-therapy-may-help-improve-womens-heart-health-overall-survival/

https://www.heartuk.org.uk/cholesterol/causes

Hypothyroidism & Hyperthyroidism

Hypothyroidism is diagnosed when the thyroid gland does not produce enough thyroid hormones, or there is an issue with the conversion. Hyperthyroidism is when the thyroid gland produces too many thyroid hormones. Autoimmune thyroiditis is when the body produces antibodies that attack the thyroid tissue. Testing, interpreting, and supporting thyroids is covered in my first book: Blood Labs 1.

There are many ways in which thyroid disorders may relate to dyslipidaemia, for example:

- Thyroid hormones affect the expression of HMG-CoA Reductase enzyme. Low thyroid hormones result in reduced cholesterol production, while raised thyroid hormones result in raised cholesterol production.

- Niemann-Pick C1-like 1 protein (NPC1L1) absorbs cholesterol in the intestines and decreases the breakdown of free fatty acids. Low levels of thyroid hormones increase the concentration of NPC1L1, leading to an increase in serum triglycerides.
- LDL receptors on the surface of the liver recognise and connect with lipoproteins containing Apo-B to remove them from the blood stream. Thyroid hormones increase these receptors, so in the case of hypothyroidism with low levels of thyroid hormones, the number of receptors is decreased, leading to an increase of lipoproteins in the bloodstream.
- Thyroid hormones influence the function of lipoprotein lipase (LPL) – low levels of thyroid hormone reduce the function of LPL

References:

https://www.ncbi.nlm.nih.gov/pmc/articles/PMC8859969/

https://pubmed.ncbi.nlm.nih.gov/6624364/

https://www.endocrineweb.com/conditions/hypothyroidism/hypothyroidism-and-cholesterol?fbclid=IwAR32StqqKl2ZJmU9KM70nQVSfZ2qafHdRvh04sgEIGC9t1q-S9tUMI2pw4A

https://www.heartuk.org.uk/cholesterol/causes

Other Endocrine Disorders

Endocrine disorders and the treatment of such disorders may alter lipid metabolism and levels of lipids in the plasma, resulting in increased or decreased risk of CVD.

I have summarised these in the table below:

	Total Cholesterol	LDL	HDL	TG	Lp(a)	Overall CVD risk
Growth Hormone Deficiency	↑	↑	↓	↑	↔	↑
Acromegaly	↓↑	↓↑	↓	↑	↑	↑
Overt Hypothyroidism	↑	↑	↔ or ↑	↔ or ↑	↑	↑
Subclinical Hypothyroidism	↔ or ↑	↔ or ↑	↔	↔ or ↑	↔	?
Hyperthyroid	↓	↓	↓	↓↑	↓	↑
Cushing's Syndrome	↑	↑	↓↑	↑	↔ or ↑	↑
Low testosterone (men)	↑	↑	↓	↑	↑	?
Androgen deprivation therapy	↑	↑	↑	↑	↑	?
Loss of oestrogens (menopause)	↔ or ↑	↑	↔ or ↓	↑	↔ or ↑	↑
PCOS	↔ or ↑	↑	↓	↑	↑	↑
Prolactinomas	↑	↑	↔ or ↓	↔ or ↓	?	↑

Table source: https://www.ncbi.nlm.nih.gov/books/NBK409608

Key:

↓ = decreased

↑ = increased

↓↑ = variable

↔ = normal or no change

? = not known

Kidney Disease

Individuals with chronic kidney disease (mild or severe) who are aged over 50 are at increased risk of CVD. The Renal Association in the UK, and the Association of Clinical Diabetologists recommend that those with kidney disease aim for total cholesterol of less than 4.0 mmol/L and LDL less than 2.0mmol/L.

- Inflammation may affect any part of the body, including arteries. Raised blood pressure (as a cause or result of chronic kidney disease) contributes to further damage of the arteries.
- Cytokines released as a response to inflammation in the body suppress appetite, leading to malnutrition. Chronic inflammation may lead to chronically high levels of cytokines and a lower intake of food/nutrients, leading to lower cholesterol overall, but also weaker muscles including the heart due to malnutrition.

Individuals with chronic kidney disease may present with raised LDL (particularly sdLDL), raised triglycerides, and low HDL. Interventions would be required to manage diet and lifestyle accordingly.

Individuals with nephrotic syndrome may present with raised cholesterol and triglycerides.

Individuals who have received a kidney transplant may have raised total cholesterol and triglycerides after the transplant due to medication side effects, weight gain, diet, immobility, or family history. Manage with diet, lifestyle as allowed post-operative, and medication as prescribed.

References

https://www.ncbi.nlm.nih.gov/pmc/articles/PMC8472557

https://www.kidney.org.uk/cholesterol-and-kidney-disease

https://www.kidney.org/atoz/content/immunosuppression

https://www.uptodate.com/contents/lipid-abnormalities-in-nephrotic-syndrome

https://www.heartuk.org.uk/cholesterol/causes

https://www.davita.com/education/kidney-disease/risk-factors/cholesterol-and-chronic-kidney-disease

Gout

Gout is a type of arthritis whereby urate crystals accumulate in the joints due to raised levels of uric acid in the blood, resulting in severe pain, swelling, redness, and tenderness in one or more joints.

Episodes can come and go suddenly, and there is an association between raised uric acid during episodes of gout and raised triglycerides.

References

https://www.heartuk.org.uk/cholesterol/causes

https://pubmed.ncbi.nlm.nih.gov/2739579/

https://www.heartuk.org.uk/cholesterol/causes

CHAPTER 10: MODIFIABLE DIET AND LIFESTYLE RISK FACTORS

These are guidelines to consider when supporting your clients with cholesterol issues – if you can address as many of these risk factors as possible, it may reduce your client's risk of atherosclerotic cardiovascular disease.

1. **Stop smoking.** There are smoking cessation services available with the NHS, or they may prefer to consider hypnotherapy, books (e.g. Allen Carr's Easy Way to Stop Smoking) or going cold turkey. Smoking increases the risk of blood clots in the blood vessels, increases blood pressure, raises oxidative stress, reduces nitric oxide in the blood vessels, reduces the amount of oxygen reaching the body tissues. In short, smoking is a major risk factor.

2. **Hydrate with water.** Avoid fizzy drinks (diet or normal) and maintain adequate hydration with filtered water. Poor hydration is one cause of raised blood pressure and raised blood pressure is a risk factor in atherosclerotic cardiovascular disease. 1-2 cups of coffee or green tea may also be beneficial in lowering cholesterol levels, but water should be the priority.

3. **Avoid frequent intake of alcohol**. Alcohol is associated with a raise in blood pressure, raise in oxidative stress, and weight gain, which would increase the risk of atherosclerotic cardiovascular disease.

4. **Avoid sugar and refined carbohydrates.** This includes excess fructose and fructose syrups. These will cause imbalances in blood glucose levels, increasing the risk of insulin resistance and inflammation. 1-2 pieces of whole fruit per day is acceptable. Aim to start each day with a savoury breakfast rather than a bowl of sweetened cereals.

5. **Reduce chemical exposure where possible.** This includes choosing fresh, ideally organic foods, over processed foods with artificial sweeteners, artificial flavours, preservatives etc. It also includes choosing personal care products with less chemicals, avoiding excessive exposure to household/industrial cleaning products and solvents, not using plastic food storage with BPA, and minimising exposure to pollution where achievable. Chemicals are inflammatory and not supportive of cardiovascular health.

6. **Prioritise sleep.** Aim for 7-8 hours of good quality sleep. Sleep deprivation is associated with an increased risk of cardiovascular disease.

7. **Daylight exposure and vitamin D.** Test vitamin D levels every 3-4 months and ensure adequate daylight exposure and/or vitamin D supplementation to maintain vitamin D levels of 90-100nmol/L. Download and use the DMinder app to check vitamin D from daylight in your client's local area, on any day.

8. **Exercise daily.** Even 30 minutes walking per day, ideally after a large meal. For those who currently do less

than this, this may reduce their risk of cardiovascular disease. For those who are already active, walking after a meal may reduce risk of insulin resistance. If you are not a personal trainer, it will be outside of your remit to recommend specific exercises. Refer your client to a personal trainer where relevant.

9. **Increase soluble fibre.** Consumed as part of a diet rich in whole grains, fruits, and vegetables, 5-10g of soluble fibre per day may reduce LDL (as well as doing wonders for bowel movements and gut health). Soluble fibre may be found in wholegrains e.g. brown rice, quinoa, oats, beans, lentils, flaxseeds, avocado, vegetables such as brussel sprouts, broccoli, carrots, green beans, and some fruits such as mango, apple, orange, peach, and berries.

10. **Introduce polyphenols.** Foods such as extra virgin olive oil, berries, cacao powder (ideally not in sugary milk chocolate!), herbs, and spices. Polyphenols work as antioxidants in the body, reducing oxidative stress and the risk of cardiovascular disease.

11. **Support nitric oxide levels.** Foods such as beetroot, leafy greens, garlic, citrus fruits, pomegranate, nuts, seeds, and watermelon may all support the production of nitric oxide in the blood vessels, essential for maintaining vascular homeostasis.

12. **Maintain a moderate intake of saturated fats.** Saturated fats will raise LDL cholesterol resulting in a

need for further exploration to ensure it is lbLDL rather than sdLDL.

13. **Consider intermittent fasting.** If appropriate for your client (e.g. no history of eating disorders, disordered eating, diabetes etc.) fasting may reduce cholesterol levels and improve insulin response.

14. **Include anti-inflammatory and/or cholesterol modifying foods:**

    a. **Nuts** – in moderation (30g per day) nuts are a natural source of plant sterols and may reduce cholesterol levels and reduce risk of complications in individuals with previous history of cardiovascular disease.

    b. **Oily fish** – a natural source of omega 3 fatty acids, known to reduce inflammation and lower blood pressure.

    c. **Avocado** – rich in monounsaturated fatty acids, one avocado per day may reduce LDL.

    d. **Extra Virgin Olive Oil** – replace all seed oils and any other processed oils with extra virgin olive oil in moderation.

    e. **Berries** – loaded with polyphenols, and sweet enough to replace the sugar removed from the diet. Anthocyanins (dark fruits and vegetables e.g. cherries, red cabbage, aubergine) help to improve insulin sensitivity.

    f. **Garlic** – epidemiological evidence supports garlic consumption for slowing progression of cardiovascular disease and reducing blood pressure.

g. **Ginger** – has anti-inflammatory properties, reduces oxidative stress, and lowers blood pressure.

h. **Whey Protein** – 20g per day added to food/drinks may lower LDL and total cholesterol, as well as blood pressure.

i. **Organic Soya Protein** – 25-50g per day may reduce LDL cholesterol levels by 4-8%.

j. **Beta-glucans** – 5g of beta-glucans a day may reduce total cholesterol by 2-5% (50g of oats contains approximately 2g of beta-glucan). Seaweed and shiitake mushrooms also contain beta-glucan.

15. Supplements (optional):

a. **Omega 3** – 3g of EPA/DHA per day, or 3g of EPA per day.

b. **Vitamin C** – 1000-2000mg per day in divided doses.

c. **B Complex** – a good quality b complex providing adequate levels of B3, B6, B9, and B12 among other b vitamins.

d. **Magnesium** – 300-600mg per day.

e. **Prebiotics and Probiotics** – at least 1bn CFU per day x 1.5 months, or milk-based kefir/yoghurt daily.

References

https://www.ncbi.nlm.nih.gov/pmc/articles/PMC2845795/

https://www.ncbi.nlm.nih.gov/pmc/articles/PMC3449318/

https://www.ahajournals.org/doi/full/10.1161/01.CIR.102.20.2555

https://pubmed.ncbi.nlm.nih.gov/27797709/

https://www.ncbi.nlm.nih.gov/pmc/articles/PMC3798856/

https://www.ncbi.nlm.nih.gov/pmc/articles/PMC3449318/

https://www.chemscape.com/resources/chemical-management/health-effects/heart-disease

https://link.springer.com/article/10.1007/s11906-020-01080-y

https://www.thelancet.com/journals/eclinm/article/PIIS2589-5370(21)00277-7/fulltext

https://pubmed.ncbi.nlm.nih.gov/26064792/

https://openheart.bmj.com/content/5/2/e000775

https://www.lipid.org/sites/default/files/adding_soluble_fiber_final_0.pdf

https://www.hopkinsmedicine.org/health/conditions-and-diseases/smoking-and-cardiovascular-disease

https://pubmed.ncbi.nlm.nih.gov/6294004/ ,

https://academic.oup.com/view-large/109820549?login=false

https://www.chhs.colostate.edu/krnc/monthly-blog/what-are-polyphenols-another-great-reason-to-eat-fruits-and-veggies

https://pubmed.ncbi.nlm.nih.gov/24034411/

https://www.nhs.uk/live-well/quit-smoking/nhs-stop-smoking-services-help-you-quit/

https://www.uscjournal.com/articles/menopause-cholesterol-and-cardiovascular-disease-0

https://pubmed.ncbi.nlm.nih.gov/29511019/

https://olivewellnessinstitute.org/article/how-does-olive-oil-compare-with-coconut-oil/

https://pubmed.ncbi.nlm.nih.gov/19115123/

https://www.mayoclinic.org/diseases-conditions/high-blood-cholesterol/in-depth/cholesterol/art-20045192

https://advances.umw.edu.pl/pdf/2018/27/1/135.pdf

https://www.ncbi.nlm.nih.gov/pmc/articles/PMC139960/

CHAPTER 11: CASE STUDY

In this chapter we are not diagnosing.

I will be presenting a mock client to you, based on a client I have been working with in my clinic since February 2022 (I have full permission to share test results). We will be looking at the client's' lipids and I will take you through how I might interpret the test results and the appropriate action to take, including further tests.

Remember, the recommendations made here are the case study. They are not for you, and not for your clients. Every case must be interpreted separately, as individuals are just that - individual. Please refer to the medical disclaimer at the beginning of the book for more details.

It is always recommended that you inform your client's doctor of your concerns, even if the doctor has previously considered the client's blood tests or symptoms to be "normal".

If you're newly qualified or not feeling 100% confident with anything covered so far in this book, please do come and join my free Facebook group www.facebook.com/groups/BloodLabs where we look at blood results and discuss how we may want to support our clients.

Initial Appointment

Synopsis

Female "SB"

Age 44

Lives in Scotland but travels regularly to warmer/sunnier climates, using SPF daily as recommended by aesthetician.

Personal trainer

Diet – Largely Paleo-style diet (meat/fish, no legumes, no refined carbohydrates) and cooking exclusively with coconut oil. Fasting most days until 1pm, drinking coffee with full-fat cow's milk while fasting.

- **Breakfast:** Fasting (coffee with cow's milk)
- **Morning snack:** Fasting (coffee with cow's milk)
- **Lunch:** Omelette with vegetables, cooked with coconut oil
- **Afternoon snack:** None
- **Evening Meal:** Meat/poultry/fish with vegetables and sweet potatoes, all cooked with coconut oil
- **Desserts:** weekends only – sticky toffee pudding etc

Consuming 15g (1 tablespoon) coconut oil per day

Drinks – water, fizzy water, herbal tea, mint tea. 3 x coffees with full fat cow's milk. No regular intake of alcohol.

Main concern: Father died of heart attack aged 56 and was diagnosed with lifestyle related atherosclerosis – smoking, drinking, vegetable oils – and SB would like to mitigate the risks associated with any hereditary conditions. Doctor has tested SB's lipid profile in past 12 months and SB is aware she has raised cholesterol and would like to clarify the numbers. Doctor has mentioned statins to lower cholesterol levels which SB won't take as she has faith in her diet and lifestyle, and would like to explore the results further. Also keen to discuss her current diet, which she has researched heavily, to see if there are any further improvements possible.

Observations:

- Height: 162cm
- Weight: 62kg
- Waist measurement: 71.2cm
- Blood pressure: unknown
- No clubbing of fingernails
- No Frank's sign (ear lobe creases)
- No obvious presence of xanthomata

Supplements: none.

Medications: none.

Red Flags: none.

Test Matrix

Looking at the Cardiovascular Testing Matrix, there are some signs that we should think about further testing. I have highlighted these on the copy of the Matrix overleaf. The rows shaded grey match SB's reported history:

- Her previous history of raised lipids
- Her family history of atherosclerotic cardiovascular disease would suggest that the full spectrum of tests available would be worth running

Initially, we agreed to review the test results from her doctor today and then select further tests, likely to be run privately, as part of our 2nd appointment.

Cardiovascular Blood Testing Matrix for SB Case Study:

	Basic Lipids Panel	Advanced Lipids Profile	HbA1C	C-Peptide	Fasting Insulin	Fasting Glucose	HS-CRP	ESR	Coronary Arterial Calcium
Aged 40+ and not aware of cholesterol levels	X		X				X	X	
Previous history of dyslipidaemia	X	X	X	X	X	X	X	X	X
Raised blood pressure	X		X				X	X	
Diagnosed with diabetes Types 1, 1.5 (LADA), or 2	X	X	X	X	X	X	X	X	
Poor eating habits	X		X	X	X	X	X	X	
Sedentary lifestyle	X		X		X	X	X	X	
Increased waist measurement	X		X	X	X	X	X	X	
Family history of dyslipidaemia	X		X				X	X	X
Family history of raised blood pressure	X		X				X	X	
Family history of cardiovascular disease	X	X	X	X	X	X	X	X	X
Clubbed fingers	X		X				X	X	
Ear lobe creasing (Frank's sign)	X		X				X	X	
Xanthomata presence	X	X	X	X	X	X	X	X	
Chronic Kidney Disease / Nephrotic Kidneys	X	X	X	X	X	X	X	X	X

Initial blood results

Marker	Result		Lab Reference Range	
Total cholesterol	6	mmol/L	0-5	↑
LDL	3.73	mmol/L	<3	↑
HDL	1.76	mmol/L	>1.2	
Non-HDL Cholesterol	4.24	mmol/L	<4	↑
Triglycerides	1.13	mmol/L	<1.7 (fasting)	
Cholesterol:HDL ratio	3.41		<4	
TG:HDL ratio	1.47			
HbA1C	29	mmol/mol	<42	
ALT	33	U/L	<35	
AST	25	U/L	<35	

Initial Thoughts

The blood results are showing raised Total Cholesterol, LDL, and non-HDL. On discussion with SB, she was unable to recall whether her test had been done in a fasted state. Fasting affects blood lipid levels (see chapter 4) so it is worth repeating the basic lipids profile to confirm raised cholesterol.

The HbA1C level is reassuringly low, but we need to establish whether large amounts of insulin are required to maintain that level of blood glucose control. Fasting glucose, fasting insulin, and C-peptide may be worthwhile tests to consider.

ALT and AST are slightly raised, but could they be raised from early insulin resistance, or perhaps from the blood test being done late in the day rather than the morning. It would be beneficial to repeat these to rule these factors out.

SB agreed to private testing options going forwards, as she would prefer an independent opinion rather than her doctor whom she feels may be biased towards prescribing statins rather than investigating further.

Estimated QRISK score: 1.6%. This is low, but only an estimate. We need further data to calculate an actual score.

Information Provided to SB following Appointment

1. We need to repeat the lipid profile (cholesterol) blood tests, but on a fasted sample. As agreed, we will test these privately, along with HbA1C, fasting insulin, fasting glucose, and C-Peptide, plus a full "MOT" to explore the fatigue in more detail. This will help us to understand the basic lipid profile in more detail.
   a. No food after midnight the night before testing
   b. No drinks after midnight the night before testing
   c. Only water can and should be consumed in the morning, prior to the test (this is important to ensure the blood draw is successful)
   d. Please avoid all supplements for at least 5 days prior to testing
2. Continue with current diet and lifestyle in the meantime

3. No other changes until bloods have been repeated

We will review your new blood results and establish required dietary/lifestyle changes at the next appointment.

1st Follow-Up Appointment

Synopsis: We had not made any changes to SB's diet following the initial appointment, so no changes in symptoms were identified at this appointment.

New blood test results

Marker	Result	Units	Lab Reference Range	
Total Cholesterol	6.27	mmol/L	0-5	↑
LDL	3.85	mmol/L	<3	↑
HDL	2.03	mmol/L	>1.2	
Non-HDL Cholesterol	4.24	mmol/L	<4	↑
Triglycerides	0.86	mmol/L	<1.7 (Fasting)	
Cholesterol:HDL ratio	3.09		<4	
TG:HDL ratio	0.96		<3	
ALT	26	U/L	<35	
Vitamin D	92	nmol/L	75-100	
HbA1C	33	mmol/mol	<42	
C-Peptide	0.58	ug/L	1.1-4.4	↓
Insulin	4.8	uIU/mL	1-15	
CRP	0.74	mg/L	<5	

Initial Thoughts

- Looking at cholesterol first, we can see that SB's total cholesterol, LDL, and non-HDL are still raised, even though this was a fasting blood test.
    - We need to investigate the LDL further, in terms of sdLDL and lbLDL breakdown, to identify if the raised LDL indicate an increased risk of atherosclerosis
- We were unable to get fasting glucose tested, so we can't calculate HOMA-IR. However, the fasting

triglycerides remain reassuringly low (as does the TG:HDL ratio), and C-peptide and fasting insulin are also reassuringly low, indicating that SB's diet is reducing the risk of insulin resistance.

- Estimated QRisk score: 1.5%. This is still an estimate, and we need to obtain further data (blood pressure) to improve accuracy of QRisk score algorithm

Information Provided to SB Following Appointment

1. Check blood pressure with your doctor or a pharmacist, or use a home blood pressure monitor, so that we can calculate your QRisk score with greater accuracy
2. Undertake a fasted Liposcan test with Nordic Laboratories, to evaluate the breakdown of sdLDL and lbLDL
   a. No food after midnight the night before testing
   b. No drinks after midnight the night before testing
   c. Only water can and should be consumed in the morning, prior to the test (this is important to ensure the blood draw is successful)
   d. Please avoid all supplements for at least 5 days prior to testing

2nd Follow-Up Appointment

Synopsis: This appointment was only a few weeks after the initial appointment, so symptoms remained as before.

Blood pressure confirmed as 119/70.

Nordic Labs Liposcan (fasted) Blood Test Results

Test	Result	Units	Lab Reference Range	
Total Cholesterol	6.75	mmol/m	<5.17	↑
Triglycerides	0.80	mmol/m	<1.7	
HDL	2.09	mmol/m	>1.16	
LDL	3.96	mmol/m	<3.36	↑
LDL:HDL	1.9		<3	
VLDL	0.72	mmol/m	<0.59	↑
IDL	0.85	mmol/m	<1.66	
Non-Pathogenic LDL subfractions				
LDL1	2.20	mmol/m	<1.5	↑
LDL2	0.85	mmol/m	<0.8	↑
Pathogenic LDL subfractions				
LDL3	0.05	mmol/m	<0.18	
LDL4	0	mmol/m	0	
LDL5	0	mmol/m	0	
LDL6	0	mmol/m	0	
LDL7	0	mmol/m	0	

Initial Thoughts

- Total cholesterol has not increased from the previous test.
- The LDL breakdown from this test is reassuring – although levels are raised overall, it is mostly lbLDL (types 1 and 2) rather than sdLDL (types 3-7).

- Actual QRisk Score: 0.8% - this is much lower than the estimated QRisk previously, and a low risk overall.
- Consider CACS for verification of low risk of atherosclerotic cardiovascular disease.
- Consider Randox Heart Panel blood test for an advanced lipids profile (currently only available in London).

Information Provided to SB following Appointment

Overall, your risk of atherosclerotic cardiovascular disease appears to be low at this time based on your LDL subtypes. Your current diet, which I know you have researched extensively, is very supportive of your cardiovascular and general health, and you should feel confident to continue eating this way as long as your lifestyle remains healthy (e.g. not smoking, not consuming excess alcohol etc)

For further reassurance, you may want to consider a coronary arterial calcium scan (CACS) to look for calcium build-up in your arteries, which would be indicative of damage and inflammation in your arteries, and your overall risk of atherosclerotic cardiovascular disease. This can is available privately from Nuffield Health, BUPA, etc.

Next time you are in London, you may also want to consider taking an advanced lipid profile blood test, such as Randox Heart Health, to evaluate your apolipoproteins and your Lp(a) levels.

As you head into perimenopause, your oestrogen levels will decline. This may result in your cholesterol levels raising even further. I would suggest monitoring your blood pressure and cholesterol levels every 6 months.

Looking at DNA, you may want to consider running a methylation panel with LifecodeGX to review your methylation genes, to ensure we are supporting your B12, folate, and homocysteine levels appropriately.

CHAPTER 11: THE CLOSING CHAPTER

My aim when writing this book was to educate you on the topic of blood tests for clients with dyslipidaemia, and/or cardiovascular risk factors, through sharing some of the research that exists on the subject.

Hopefully, you are now feeling more confident and more prepared for your next client and will be ready to interpret their cholesterol panel blood results or request new blood tests if needed.

The case study used in this book is useful, but it is not specific to you or your clients.

Every set of blood tests that your client has will need to be researched, considered in context, and acted upon appropriately – one person's raised LDL may be caused by something entirely different to the next persons.

If you've found this book useful, please do consider leaving an honest review on Amazon for others to read, and if you haven't purchased copies already, then I also have two other books available on Amazon, covering blood test interpretation for fatigue, and hormones.

If you're still finding the subject of blood test interpretation confusing or overwhelming, or you're feeling less than confident, you are more than welcome to contact me, and we can discuss the subject in more detail. For this, please email clinic@kateknowler.co.uk and we can discuss your options for a strategic mentoring session with myself.

Also, don't forget that I also have my TOTALLY FREE Facebook group which you are welcome to join if you haven't already, in which I provide free support for you with blood test interpretation.

I'm here to help you!

Kate xx

Facebook group: Blood Test Interpretation with Kate Knowler

Book 1: Blood Labs – A Guide to Interpreting Blood Test Results for Fatigue

Book 2: Blood Labs – A Guide to Interpreting Blood Test Results for Hormones

Email: clinic@kateknowler.co.uk

Additional references used throughout this book:

Put Your Heart in Your Mouth – Dr. Natasha Campbell

The Great Cholesterol Con – Dr. Malcolm Kendrick

A Statin Free Life – Dr. Aseem Malhotra

What Your Doctor May Not Tell You About Heart Disease – Dr. Mark Houston

Cholesterol Clarity – Jimmy Moore

Printed in Great Britain
by Amazon

45849490R00089